SUN TZU
The Art of War For Health & Longevity

The Warrior's Way to Wellness

Y. TONY YANG

TUTTLE Publishing

Tokyo | Rutland, Vermont | Singapore

To Katie, Avery, Linus, and Cason—my steadfast allies in life's campaign—who remind me daily that our greatest strategic victory lies in love freely given.

Contents

Preface.. 5

Introduction: The Warrior's Path to Wellness 9

Chapter 1	Laying Plans: Building Your Health Strategy 21
Chapter 2	Mastering Health: The Economics of Wellness Maintenance 39
Chapter 3	Attack by Stratagem: Winning with Preventive Measures 55
Chapter 4	Tactical Dispositions: Positioning Yourself for Health Success 73
Chapter 5	Energy: Harnessing Your Inner Strength ... 87
Chapter 6	Weak Points and Strong: Recognizing and Overcoming Vulnerabilities................. 101
Chapter 7	Maneuvering: Navigating the Challenges of Daily Health............................... 123
Chapter 8	Variation in Tactics: Flexibility in Health Strategies............................ 139
Chapter 9	The Body on the March: Guiding Your Physical Journey 155
Chapter 10	Terrain: Understanding the Health Landscape........................... 173

Chapter 11 The Nine Situations: Facing Various
            Health Challenges *193*

Chapter 12 The Attack by Fire: Targeted Actions for
            Health Breakthroughs *211*

Chapter 13 The Use of Intelligence: Monitoring and
            Learning from Your Health *229*

The Way Ahead: Surrendering to Victory *247*

Author's Notes *255*

Preface

The ancient text rested in my hands, characters dancing across rice paper like black ants forming battle formations. I was eight, sitting cross-legged on the floor of my father's study in Taipei, struggling to decipher the classical Chinese of *The Art of War*. The language was simultaneously familiar and foreign—my native tongue, yet rendered in its ancient form, dense with meanings that shifted like shadows as my understanding deepened.

"知彼知己，百戰不殆," my father read aloud. "Know the enemy and know yourself, and in a hundred battles you will never be in peril."

He paused, eyes twinkling behind wire-rimmed glasses. "But what is your greatest enemy, and what does it mean to truly know yourself?"

This question echoed through decades as my path carried me from the narrow lanes of Taipei to the sprawling campuses of American universities, eventually leading to my current position as a tenured Professor of Health Policy. The journey transformed me in ways both profound and subtle—language, culture, perspective—yet Sun Tzu's wisdom remained a constant companion, a philosophical touchstone that bridged Eastern and Western worldviews.

What I could not have anticipated as that curious child was how profoundly Master Sun's military strategy would illuminate the battlefields of human health. The parallels revealed themselves gradually, first as intellectual curiosity, then as compelling framework, and finally as the organizing principle for this book.

Health, I came to realize, represents the most intimate terrain of conflict we will ever navigate. The strategies we deploy—or fail to deploy—determine not just longevity but the quality of our existence. Yet Western medicine often approaches this campaign with tactical fragmentation rather than strategic coherence, treating symptoms while overlooking the integrated systems where both disease and wellness originate.

This book emerges from the unique vantage point of someone who straddles worlds: Eastern and Western, ancient wisdom and modern science, philosophical tradition and empirical research. The text you hold represents neither pure Eastern mysticism nor clinical Western pragmatism, but rather a synthesis born of cultural fluency in both realms.

When I speak of "water flowing downhill" as metaphor for effortless health strategies, I draw not from superficial appropriation but from cultural inheritance—memories of mountain streams in Taiwan's misty highlands and late-night discussions of Taoist principles with village elders. When I reference randomized controlled trials or health policy frameworks, I speak with the authority of academic rigor and years navigating America's complex healthcare landscape.

The Art of War for Health and Longevity does not claim to resolve the tensions between traditional wisdom and modern medicine. Rather, it acknowledges these apparent contradictions as complementary forces that, properly harmonized, create something greater than either could achieve alone—much like the concept of *yin* and *yang* that informed Sun Tzu's own strategic thinking.

As you journey through these pages, you will encounter principles that have survived twenty-five centuries not because they offer quick solutions or miraculous cures, but because they reveal enduring truths about strategy, adaptation, and the nature of conflict itself. Whether facing cancer, chronic disease, aging, or simply the daily challenge of maintaining vitality in our modern environment, these ancient insights illuminate paths forward that neither blind adherence to tradition nor uncritical faith in technology can provide alone.

In the classical Chinese tradition, the true mark of wisdom is not in knowing many things, but in recognizing the patterns that connect seemingly disparate domains of knowledge. It is my hope that this work honors that tradition while serving the very practical purpose of guiding you through the most important campaign you will ever wage—the one for your own health and vitality.

The warrior who truly understands strategy knows that the greatest victory requires no battle at all. Perhaps, in health as in warfare, the supreme achievement lies not in treating disease once it manifests, but in creating conditions where illness struggles to establish itself in the first place.

To your strategic health,
Y. Tony Yang

Introduction: The Warrior's Path to Wellness

The doctor's office was sterile and cold. John sat on the examination table, the paper crinkling beneath him with every anxious shift. Three specialists, seven prescriptions, and thousands of dollars later, he was no closer to understanding why he felt so persistently unwell. "Take these pills," they said. "Lose some weight. Come back in six months." Each interaction brief, impersonal—a transaction rather than a transformation.[1]

This scene repeats countless times daily across the modern world—a world where our approach to health has become as fragmented as our lives. We treat symptoms, not systems. We react to illness rather than cultivating wellness. We surrender our most precious asset—our health—to institutions and "experts" who know our lab results but not our lives.

This is not a criticism of modern medicine—its miracles are undeniable. This is a wake-up call about our relationship with our own bodies.

The Battle We're Losing

In the sleek corridors of our technological age, an invisible war rages. The statistics speak volumes: chronic diseases—heart disease, diabetes, cancer—now account for 7 of 10 deaths in America. Autoimmune disorders affect 50 million Americans. Mental health conditions burden one in five adults. Meanwhile, we've witnessed global vulnerabilities exposed by pandemics, revealing how unprepared our systems—and our bodies—are for unexpected threats.

This isn't merely a healthcare crisis. It's a crisis of perspective.

We approach our bodies as machines that occasionally malfunction, requiring technical repairs. We separate physical health from mental wellbeing, nutrition from movement, medical interventions from daily habits. We've embraced a transactional model of health: you get sick, you pay for treatment, you move on—until the next crisis.

This approach is failing us.

Consider Emma, a corporate executive who, at 42, seemed to "have it all"—except health. Her medicine cabinet resembled a small pharmacy: pills for sleep, for anxiety, for acid reflux, for headaches. Her schedule allowed no space for proper meals or movement. Her doctor appointments were rushed affairs, addressing each symptom separately. When COVID-19 struck, her compromised immune system left her battling long-term complications. "No one ever taught me to think about my health as a connected system," she later reflected. "I treated my body like a reluctant servant rather than an ally."

Emma's story isn't unique. It's emblematic of our collective misunderstanding.

The Call for Radical Rethinking

Two and a half millennia ago, Sun Tzu wrote, "The supreme art of war is to subdue the enemy without fighting." This ancient wisdom holds the key to a revolutionary approach to health. What if we stopped fighting against our bodies and started fighting *for* them? What if wellness wasn't a series of isolated battles against symptoms but a strategic campaign for vitality?

This book is born from necessity. We need a new paradigm—not because modern medicine has failed, but because our relationship with it is incomplete. *The Art of War for Health and Longevity* proposes a radical rethinking: your body is not a battlefield where you wage war against disease, but a kingdom you must wisely govern and protect.

Consider these fundamental shifts:

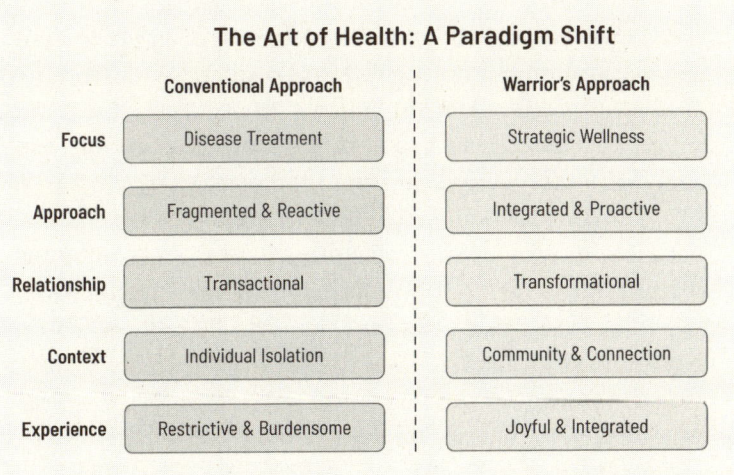

From Fragmentation to Integration: Your body doesn't recognize the artificial boundaries between "digestive health"

and "mental health." Your immune system doesn't separate "stress management" from "nutrition." Everything connects. When Michael, a 35-year-old teacher, addressed his chronic digestive issues, he was surprised when his anxiety diminished simultaneously. His doctors had treated these as separate conditions for years. Only when he adopted an integrated approach—acknowledging how sleep affected his gut, how gut health affected his mind—did he begin to heal.

From Transaction to Transformation: Health is not something you purchase at the pharmacy or the gym. It's something you cultivate, day by day, choice by choice. When Sofia, recovering from heart surgery at 51, shifted from asking "which pill can fix this?" to "how can I redesign my life to support my heart?," everything changed. Her recovery wasn't merely medical; it was personal, environmental, and spiritual.

From Isolation to Community: The Western ideal of self-reliance has infiltrated our health model, leaving us to navigate complex systems alone. Yet humans evolved to heal in community. Research shows that strong social connections can improve recovery rates and reduce mortality risk by up to 50%. When David created a "health council" of friends who walked with him, cooked with him, and held him accountable after his diabetes diagnosis, his health markers improved more significantly than those of patients who relied solely on medical intervention.

From Drudgery to Joy: We've accepted the narrative that healthy living equals restriction—joyless salads and punishing exercise. This perspective virtually guarantees failure. What if health-supporting habits could be the most pleasurable parts of your day? When Leila redesigned her fitness routine around dance—which she loved—rather than the gym work she dreaded, her consistency increased tenfold. When Marcus discovered that his Mediterranean heritage offered delicious ways to eat anti-inflammatory foods, healthy eating became a celebration rather than a sentence.

The COVID-19 pandemic revealed how unprepared we were—not just in our healthcare systems, but in our personal health strategies. Those with robust preventive health practices and strong immune systems often fared better. The crisis underscored that waiting for illness to strike before taking action isn't just risky; it can be fatal.

Sun Tzu wrote: "Victorious warriors win first and then go to war, while defeated warriors go to war first and then seek to win." In health terms, the victorious don't wait for disease to declare war on their bodies. They prepare the terrain so thoroughly that many battles never materialize.

The Warrior's Approach to Health

In Sun Tzu's world, a general's wisdom was measured not by the battles won, but by the battles made unnecessary through strategy and preparation. Similarly, your health wisdom should be judged not by how many illnesses you've overcome, but by how many you've prevented through mindful living.

This requires the mindset of a warrior: disciplined but flexible, strategic but adaptable, fierce but patient. The warrior knows when to advance and when to retreat, when to use force and when to yield. Most importantly, the warrior understands that strength comes not just from weapons but from wisdom.

I witnessed this warrior spirit in Sara, diagnosed with rheumatoid arthritis at 29. Rather than surrendering to a lifetime of increasing medication and declining mobility, she researched extensively, assembled a diverse team of health allies, eliminated inflammatory triggers from her environment, adopted meditation for stress management, and completely redesigned her nutrition and movement patterns. Five years later, her disease markers had improved so dramatically that her rheumatologist used her case in teaching. "I didn't just treat my arthritis," Sara explained. "I created conditions where it couldn't thrive."

This isn't magical thinking. It's strategy.

When Sun Tzu wrote about knowing yourself and knowing your enemy, he could have been describing Sara's approach. She learned her genetic predispositions, her specific inflammatory triggers, her unique responses to different foods and movements. She studied her "enemy"—rheumatoid arthritis—understanding its mechanisms, its patterns, its vulnerabilities. Armed with this knowledge, she fought not with desperation but with precision.

Why This Book Now?

We stand at a critical juncture in human health. Our technological advancement has far outpaced our health wisdom. We can map the human genome but struggle to maintain basic wellness. We can perform miraculous surgeries but can't seem to prevent the conditions that make them necessary.

The statistics are alarming:
- 60% of Americans have at least one chronic condition
- 88% show signs of metabolic dysfunction
- Anxiety and depression have increased 25% worldwide since the pandemic
- Autoimmune disorders are increasing at rates that cannot be explained by genetics alone

The conventional approach isn't working because it addresses symptoms rather than systems, reactions rather than prevention, illness rather than wellness. We need a new blueprint.

The Art of War for Health and Longevity offers that blueprint, drawing wisdom from an unexpected source. Sun Tzu's strategic brilliance wasn't limited to battlefields. His understanding of human nature, systemic thinking, and strategic preparation transcends context. Applied to health, his principles offer revolutionary insights for our modern struggles.

Consider his famous counsel: "In the midst of chaos, there is also opportunity." The chaos of our current health landscape—with its contradictory advice, complex systems, and competing interests—contains the opportunity for personal empowerment. When Raj, overwhelmed by contradictory advice after his pre-diabetes diagnosis, applied Sun Tzu's principle of strategic clarity, he focused only on the changes with the highest impact: intermittent fasting, strength training, and stress reduction. Within six months, his markers normalized.

Or consider Sun Tzu's wisdom: "The greatest victory is that which requires no battle." James, who watched his father die young from heart disease, embodied this principle by creating living conditions that made heart disease unlikely: a home in a walkable neighborhood, a social life centered around active pursuits rather than sedentary dining, and cooking methods that celebrated heart-supporting ingredients. At 72, his cardiovascular health exceeds that of many 40-year-olds.

These aren't anomalies. They represent what's possible when we approach health as Sun Tzu approached warfare—with respect, strategy, and holistic thinking.

A New Vision for Health Engagement

This book envisions health not as a battlefield where you fight against disease, but as a garden you mindfully cultivate. It's not about isolated skirmishes against symptoms but about creating an ecosystem where wellness naturally flourishes.

This means:
- Treating your body not as a machine to be repaired but as a complex, intelligent system to be supported
- Viewing health professionals not as mechanics who fix you but as allies who guide you
- Considering food not as fuel to be calculated but as information that speaks directly to your genes
- Approaching movement not as punishment for calories consumed but as a celebration of what your body can do
- Recognizing stress not as an inevitable byproduct of modern life but as a strategic vulnerability to be addressed
- Understanding sleep not as a luxury to be sacrificed but as the foundation upon which all health is built

Most importantly, it means acknowledging that true health emerges not from isolated interventions but from the thousands of small choices that shape your daily life—choices about what you eat, how you move, whom you connect with, how you respond to stress, and the environments you create around yourself.

The Journey Ahead

As you make your way through this guide, you'll discover that Sun Tzu's strategic principles translate powerfully to personal wellness. You'll learn to assess your health terrain, identify vulnerabilities before they become problems, build resilience against potential threats, and respond strategically when challenges arise.

The pages ahead offer not just theory but practical application—specific strategies, actionable steps, and real-world examples drawn from both ancient wisdom and cutting-edge research. You'll meet people who have employed these principles to transform not just their physical health but their entire relationship with wellness.

The journey begins with understanding—understanding your unique body, your specific risks, your personal health landscape. It continues with strategy—developing a comprehensive approach that addresses every aspect of wellness, from nutrition and movement to stress management and environmental factors. And it culminates in implementation—turning knowledge into action, strategy into habit, information into transformation.

Your Roadmap Through the Book

This book follows the structure of Sun Tzu's original masterpiece, reimagining each chapter for the health warrior:

1. **Laying Plans: Building Your Health Strategy**—Here we'll assess your personal health landscape, examining how Sun Tzu's five pillars translate to wellness fundamentals: nutrition, exercise, mental wellbeing, environment, and preventive care.
2. **Mastering Health: The Economics of Wellness Maintenance**—We'll explore the strategic investment of resources—time, money, energy—to prevent illness and build resilience, applying Sun Tzu's principles of efficiency and effectiveness.

3. **Attack by Stratagem: Winning with Preventive Measures**—This chapter reveals how to deploy preventive strategies like screenings, vaccinations, and lifestyle interventions to outmaneuver disease before it strikes.
4. **Tactical Dispositions: Positioning Yourself for Health Success**—Learn to position yourself optimally in your lifestyle choices, creating systems that naturally support wellness rather than undermining it.
5. **Energy: Harnessing Your Inner Strength**—Discover how to cultivate and direct your motivation, willpower, and creativity to sustain healthy habits when enthusiasm wanes.
6. **Weak Points and Strong: Recognizing and Overcoming Vulnerabilities**—Identify your unique health vulnerabilities—whether genetic, environmental, or behavioral—and learn to strengthen these potential points of attack.
7. **Maneuvering: Navigating the Challenges of Daily Health**—Master the art of navigating real-world health challenges, from social pressures to time constraints, applying Sun Tzu's principles of adaptability and strategic timing.
8. **Variation in Tactics: Flexibility in Health Strategies**—Learn to adapt your health approach as conditions change, avoiding rigid adherence to outdated methods in favor of evolving, evidence-based practices.
9. **The Body on the March: Guiding Your Physical Journey**—Understand how movement shapes health outcomes and learn to deploy different forms of physical activity for specific wellness objectives.
10. **Terrain: Understanding the Health Landscape**—Explore how your environment—physical, social, and cultural—shapes your health possibilities, and learn to modify your terrain for optimal wellness.

11. **The Nine Situations: Facing Various Health Challenges**—Master strategies for different health scenarios, from preventing illness to managing chronic conditions to recovering from acute health crises.
12. **The Attack by Fire: Targeted Actions for Health Breakthroughs**—Discover when and how to deploy intensive interventions—from medical treatments to radical lifestyle changes—for maximum impact.
13. **The Use of Intelligence: Monitoring and Learning From Your Health**—Learn to gather, interpret, and apply personal health data to refine your strategies continuously, using both technology and intuition.

Each chapter blends ancient wisdom with modern science, philosophical insight with practical application, strategic thinking with daily habits. Together, they form a comprehensive approach to health that honors both the complexity of the human body and the simplicity of natural living.

As Sun Tzu might say, the greatest health victory is not overcoming disease but creating conditions where disease cannot take hold. This book will show you how to achieve that victory, day by day, choice by choice, strategy by strategy.

Your campaign for vibrant health begins now. Arm yourself with knowledge, prepare your terrain, know your vulnerabilities, and advance with both courage and wisdom. The art of health awaits.

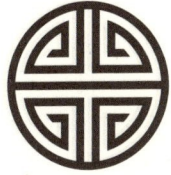

1

Laying Plans: Building Your Health Strategy

The Battlefield Within

Lisa stared at the array of pill bottles lined up on her bathroom counter like silent sentinels. Statins for cholesterol. Beta-blockers for hypertension. Sleep aids for insomnia. Anti-inflammatories for joint pain. At 43, her medicine cabinet had become a chemical arsenal against an enemy she couldn't see but felt advancing daily.

"When did my body become the battlefield?" she whispered to her reflection.

The question lingered, unanswered, as she swallowed her morning regimen.

We are all Lisa, in one way or another. Our bodies—once playgrounds, then productive machines—eventually become terrains where invisible wars are waged. Yet unlike traditional battlefields, we are simultaneously the land being fought over, the general directing troops, and the nation whose future hangs in the balance.

Sun Tzu, the legendary Chinese military strategist, wrote in *The Art of War*: "The general who wins a battle makes many calculations in his temple before the battle is fought." This ancient wisdom offers profound guidance for modern health warriors. Before we can fight effectively for our well-being, we must make our calculations—understand our terrain, assess our resources, recognize our vulnerabilities, and develop strategies that play to our strengths.

In this age of medical miracles, we've become adept at fighting disease once it arrives but woefully unprepared at preventing its advance. We deploy surgical strikes against tumors but neglect the daily skirmishes that determine whether those tumors form. We marshal pharmaceutical troops against heart disease but ignore the supply lines of nutrition that feed it. We've become reactive generals waiting for the enemy to breach our walls rather than proactive strategists securing our borders.

This chapter is your war council. Here, we will learn to think like health strategists rather than medical tacticians. We will develop not just a battle plan but a campaign strategy—comprehensive, personalized, and adaptable.

Reconnoitering Your Personal Health Landscape

Consider James, a 52-year-old construction manager. After his father died of a heart attack at 56, James approached his doctor with a simple question: "Am I next?" The doctor ran tests, noted James's slightly elevated blood pressure and borderline cholesterol, prescribed a mild statin, and suggested he "watch what he eats and try to exercise more."

James followed the advice half-heartedly for a few months before the pressures of work and family pushed health concerns to the background. Three years later, chest pains sent him to the emergency room. The diagnosis: severe coronary artery disease requiring immediate intervention.

"But I did what the doctor said," James protested as they prepped him for surgery.

James's mistake wasn't in failing to follow medical advice. It was in misunderstanding the nature of the battle. He had treated health as a series of disconnected skirmishes rather than a coordinated campaign. He had failed to reconnoiter his personal health landscape.

Sun Tzu teaches: "Know the enemy and know yourself; in a hundred battles you will never be in peril." In health terms, this means understanding both disease mechanisms and your unique vulnerabilities to them.

Consider how different James's story might have been if he had mapped his health landscape comprehensively:

Genetic Intelligence: Beyond knowing his father died young of heart disease, James might have explored his genetic predispositions through testing. Research shows that individuals with a family history of premature heart disease face a 50-200% increased risk of developing cardiovascular disease, depending on the closeness of the affected relative and the age at which the condition occurred.[1] Knowledge of specific genetic markers could have alerted him to particular pathways of vulnerability—inflammation, lipid metabolism, or endothelial function—each requiring different preventive strategies.

Physiological Reconnaissance: Rather than accepting "slightly elevated" numbers, James could have investigated deeper markers of cardiovascular health: inflammatory indicators like high-sensitivity C-reactive protein (which predicts cardiovascular events independent of cholesterol), lipoprotein(a) levels (a hereditary risk factor unaffected by statins), or coronary calcium scores (which show actual arterial plaque buildup). Studies demonstrate that these specialized tests can identify high-risk individuals who appear "normal" on standard screenings.

Lifestyle Analysis: James's construction job provided physical activity but also exposed him to environmental toxins and chronic stress—both significant contributors to heart disease. A comprehensive assessment would have mapped his sleep patterns (research shows that poor sleep increases cardiovascular mortality by 45%), stress management techniques, nutritional habits, and environmental exposures.

Psychological Terrain: The mind-body connection isn't metaphysical philosophy; it's biological reality. James's tendency toward perfectionism and his stoic approach to emotional challenges created patterns of chronic stress that directly impacted his cardiovascular function. Research shows that psychological factors like depression can increase the risk of heart attack by approximately 64%, while chronic stress activates inflammatory pathways that accelerate atherosclerosis.[2]

The terrain is complex. The general who fails to map it thoroughly marches blindly into battle.

The Five Pillars of Strategic Health

In *The Art of War*, Sun Tzu outlines five factors that determine military outcomes: moral law, heaven, earth, the commander, and method and discipline. These ancient pillars translate remarkably well to modern health strategy.

1. Moral Law: Core Values and Nutritional Philosophy

Sun Tzu's "moral law" refers to that which causes people to be in accord with their leader. In health terms, this represents your core values and nutritional philosophy—the principles that guide your daily choices and create internal harmony rather than conflict.

Consider Sophia, a 38-year-old marketing executive constantly cycling through diet plans. Paleo one month, vegan the next, then keto, then Mediterranean. Each plan brought temporary results followed by rebound weight gain and increasing frustration.

During a wellness retreat, a nutritionist asked her a question no one had posed before: "What food philosophy aligns with your deepest values?"

The query sparked revelation. Sophia realized her Puerto Rican heritage, environmentalist beliefs, and desire for communal eating experiences were constantly at war with whatever diet she adopted. Her breakthrough came not from finding the "perfect" diet but from developing nutritional principles aligned with her values: locally-sourced foods when possible, plant-forward but not plant-exclusive, meals that could be shared family-style, and dishes that honored her cultural traditions while adapting them for modern nutritional knowledge.

Within six months, Sophia lost 27 pounds (12.3 kilograms) without "dieting." More importantly, her inflammatory markers improved, her energy stabilized, and food became a source of joy rather than anxiety. By aligning her nutrition with her moral law, she created internal harmony that made healthy choices sustainable.

This alignment is powerful medicine. Studies show that when health behaviors connect to personal values, adherence increases by up to 73%.[3] Research reports that adults consuming adequate fruits and vegetables (at least 2 cups of fruit and 2.5 cups of vegetables daily) reduce their risk of chronic diseases by 30%—but only 10% of Americans meet these guidelines, largely because their food choices conflict with, rather than support, their values.

Your moral law might prioritize environmental sustainability, animal welfare, cultural heritage, religious practices, or family traditions. The specific values matter less than their authenticity to you and your commitment to nutritional choices that honor them.

2. Heaven: Environmental Factors and Biological Rhythms

Sun Tzu included "heaven" among his five factors, referring to seasons, weather, and timing. For health strategists, this translates to understanding both external environmental influences and internal biological rhythms.

Mark, a 45-year-old software developer in Seattle, battled seasonal depression for years. Each winter brought weight gain, lethargy, and impaired glucose regulation. His doctor prescribed antidepressants, which helped his mood but did nothing for his physical symptoms.

A functional medicine practitioner helped Mark map his "heaven" factors: the significant reduction in light exposure during Pacific Northwest winters, disruption of his circadian rhythms from blue light exposure through constant screen time, indoor air pollution from his aging apartment building, and seasonal variations in his vitamin D levels.

His personalized strategy addressed these specific environmental challenges: a therapeutic light box used for 30 minutes each morning, blue-light blocking glasses after sunset, an air purification system, and carefully timed vitamin D supplementation. He also restructured his work schedule to allow for a midday walk, regardless of weather, to ensure some exposure to natural light.

Within one winter season, Mark's transformation was remarkable. His mood stabilized without medication, his weight remained constant, and his fasting glucose levels normalized. By respecting heaven's influence—adapting to seasonal realities rather than fighting against them—he converted environmental challenges into strategic advantages.

Research confirms that light therapy is as effective as medication for seasonal mood disorders, while studies demonstrate that circadian rhythm alignment improves virtually every biomarker of health, from insulin sensitivity to immune function.[4]

Your "heaven" factors include:
- Geographic location and climate influences
- Seasonal patterns affecting your health
- Light exposure and its impact on circadian rhythms
- Air and water quality in your environment
- Technological influences on your biological functions
- Timing of meals, exercise, and sleep relative to your personal chronobiology

The general who ignores these factors fights not only disease but nature itself—a battle rarely won.

3. Earth: Physical Body and Movement Practices

Sun Tzu's "earth" encompasses the physical terrain on which battles are fought—distances, dangers, and opportunities presented by the landscape. In health, your physical body is this terrain, with its unique strengths, limitations, and optimal movement patterns.

Elena, a 36-year-old accountant, had internalized the "no pain, no gain" approach to fitness. Despite recurring injuries, she pushed through high-intensity workouts because they burned maximum calories. When persistent knee pain finally forced her to see an orthopedic specialist, she learned she had structural issues that made her chosen exercises actively harmful.

Working with a corrective exercise specialist, Elena mapped her physical terrain accurately for the first time: hypermobile joints that required stabilization rather than stretching, muscle imbalances from years at a desk, and movement patterns optimized for her particular skeletal structure.

Her revised strategy abandoned generic workout plans in favor of terrain-appropriate movement: stability training before mobility work, carefully designed strength exercises respecting her joint architecture, and low-impact cardiovascular options that built fitness without further damage.

Within three months, Elena's chronic pain subsided. More surprisingly, her body composition improved more rapidly with these personalized, moderate approaches than it had with her previous high-intensity regimen. By respecting her "earth"—working with her body's actual nature rather than her idealized vision of it—she turned apparent limitations into sustainable advantages.

The research supporting this terrain-specific approach is compelling. Studies found that exercise programs customized to individual biomechanics produced 54% better results with 67% fewer injuries compared to standardized protocols.[5] Meanwhile, research confirms that moderate exercise performed consistently yields better long-term health outcomes than sporadic intense training.

Your "earth" assessment includes:
- Structural considerations (joint structure, spinal alignment, etc.)
- Movement patterns and biomechanical efficiency
- Current fitness baselines across various modalities
- Injury history and compensatory patterns

- Recovery capacity and signals
- Body composition and metabolic response to different movement types

The wise general fights on favorable terrain. In health, this means moving in ways that respect your body's actual nature, not punishing it for failing to be something it isn't.

4. The Commander: Mental Resilience and Decision-Making

Sun Tzu placed enormous emphasis on the commander's qualities: wisdom, sincerity, benevolence, courage, and strictness. In your health campaign, you are the commander, and your mental approach determines success or failure more surely than any other factor.

Consider David, a 58-year-old professor diagnosed with type 2 diabetes. His initial response was to oscillate between denial and despair—ignoring dietary recommendations one week, then attempting unsustainable restrictions the next. His glucose levels remained dangerously high despite medication.

Working with a health psychologist, David realized his "commander problem" was approaching diabetes as a punishment rather than a strategic challenge. He was either giving orders his "troops" couldn't follow or abandoning leadership entirely.

His transformation began when he developed the five commander qualities in his approach to health:

- Wisdom: Educating himself about glucose regulation beyond simplistic rules
- Sincerity: Acknowledging his actual food preferences and habits rather than making promises he couldn't keep
- Benevolence: Treating his body with compassion rather than criticism
- Courage: Facing difficult lifestyle changes without minimizing or catastrophizing

- Strictness: Establishing clear, non-negotiable protocols for situations he knew were problematic

Six months later, David's HbA1c had dropped from 8.9% to 6.2%—nearly normal range. His medication requirements decreased by half, and his energy level soared. By addressing the commander element of his health strategy, he converted what had felt like an overwhelming defeat into a series of manageable, often rewarding, tactical adjustments.

Research shows that psychological factors predict treatment adherence more accurately than knowledge or access to care. Meanwhile, research found that patients who develop "health leadership skills," such as self-efficacy, goal-setting, and problem-solving, are significantly more likely to sustain long-term lifestyle changes compared to those who rely solely on behavioral techniques.

Your commander assessment includes:
- Decision-making patterns around health
- Emotional regulation strategies
- Self-efficacy and health locus of control
- Stress management techniques
- Cognitive patterns that help or hinder health behaviors
- Motivational clarity and personal authority

The greatest general leads neither through tyranny nor abdication but through strategic clarity and earned authority. Your body's troops respond similarly.

5. Method and Discipline: Routines and Preventive Practice

Sun Tzu's final factor—method and discipline—concerns organization, resource management, and controlled execution. In health terms, this manifests as your systems, routines, and preventive practices.

Michael, a 49-year-old airline pilot with an inherently disruptive schedule, struggled with consistent health habits.

Crossing time zones regularly made conventional routines impossible, and his health suffered accordingly—weight gain, disturbed sleep, and digestive problems became his constant companions.

Rather than attempting to impose a normal schedule on his abnormal life, Michael developed what he called "situational routines"—methodical systems that could adapt to changing conditions while maintaining essential health inputs. He created distinct protocols for home days, flight days, and layover days, each designed to provide the nutrition, movement, sleep support, and stress management appropriate to that context.

He established non-negotiable preventive practices: quarterly blood work to catch biomarker shifts early, therapeutic massage to counteract the physical strain of flying, and regular sauna sessions to support detoxification and cardiovascular health.

Within a year, despite maintaining the same challenging career, Michael reversed his health decline. His preventive approach identified a developing thyroid issue before symptoms became apparent, allowing for early intervention. His weight stabilized, his sleep quality improved despite irregular hours, and his previously concerning inflammatory markers normalized.

Evidence supports this methodical approach to chaotic circumstances. Research demonstrates that individuals with "high lifestyle irregularity" who implement context-specific health routines show significantly better health outcomes than those attempting to force standardized regimens onto irregular lives.[6] Meanwhile, preventive screenings tailored to personal risk factors can significantly reduce mortality from chronic diseases, with some studies showing reductions of up to 60% in specific high-risk populations.

Your method and discipline assessment includes:
- Systems for maintaining health inputs amid life's variability
- Routines that support rather than fight your natural inclinations
- Preventive screening schedule based on personal risk factors
- Resource allocation (time, money, attention) toward health priorities
- Feedback mechanisms to evaluate strategy effectiveness
- Contingency planning for predictable health challenges

The disciplined general anticipates challenges rather than merely reacting to them. Your health strategy requires the same forward-thinking preparation.

The Holistic Campaign: Integration Over Isolation

Sun Tzu's genius lay not in mastering individual factors but in understanding their interdependence. "The five factors are not separate matters," he wrote. "The wise general sees them as a single integrated reality."

This holistic perspective transforms health strategy from a collection of isolated interventions to an integrated campaign where each element strengthens the others.

Consider Rachel, a 41-year-old attorney whose disjointed approach to health resembled a poorly coordinated military operation. She ate "clean" but slept poorly. She exercised intensely but under chronic stress. She meditated regularly but exposed herself to environmental toxins through poorly chosen household products. Her health improvements remained frustratingly limited despite considerable effort.

Working with an integrative medicine team, Rachel learned to see these elements as interconnected fronts in a single campaign. She discovered how her high-intensity exercise was exacerbating her sleep problems, how her clean diet lacked specific nutrients that supported stress resilience, and how her meditation practice—while valuable—couldn't fully counteract the inflammatory effects of her toxic exposures.

Her revised strategy coordinated these elements: exercise timed and structured to support rather than disrupt sleep cycles, nutritional adjustments targeted to her specific stress physiology, environmental modifications that reduced her toxic burden, and mind-body practices that supported her particular nervous system patterns.

Within three months, Rachel experienced what she called a "quantum improvement"—far greater than the sum of the individual changes would suggest. Her inflammatory markers dropped significantly, her sleep efficiency improved by 62%, her stress resilience (measured by heart rate variability) increased, and her long-standing digestive issues resolved.

This integrated approach reflects cutting-edge understanding of human physiology. Research demonstrates that health outcomes emerge from complex network effects rather than linear pathways, highlighting the interconnected nature of biological systems. Studies also show that patients receiving coordinated, multi-domain interventions experience significantly better outcomes—often several times greater—compared to those receiving equally intensive but uncoordinated care, underscoring the effectiveness of holistic, systems-based approaches.

Your holistic campaign planning includes:
- Mapping the relationships between different health domains
- Identifying synergistic interventions that address multiple factors

- Recognizing compensatory patterns that undermine progress
- Coordinating timing of different health practices for maximum effect
- Balancing resource allocation across interdependent systems
- Developing metrics that capture overall health status, not isolated markers

The masterful general coordinates all elements of warfare into a unified campaign. Your body responds to the same strategic harmony.

Long-Term Victory: The Art of Sustainable Health

"There is no instance of a country having benefited from prolonged warfare," Sun Tzu observed. Yet modern health approaches often resemble endless conflicts—perpetual dieting, punishing exercise regimens, chronic medication dependencies—that deplete resources without securing lasting peace.

The art of health, like the art of war, ultimately aims not for perpetual conflict but for sustainable victory—a state where wellbeing emerges naturally from the terrain you've established rather than requiring constant battle.

Alex, a 47-year-old retail manager, epitomized the warfare approach to health. Twenty-five years of yo-yo dieting, extreme fitness phases followed by complete abandonment, periodic "detox" programs followed by binge behaviors—all had left him exhausted, cynical, and paradoxically less healthy than when he started.

His transformation began when a health coach asked a simple question: "What if health wasn't something you fought for but something you grew?"

This agricultural metaphor—health as cultivation rather

than combat—sparked a profound shift in Alex's approach. Instead of declaring war on his body's tendencies, he began working with them. Rather than pursuing quick victories through extreme measures, he focused on establishing conditions where health naturally flourished.

He replaced his all-or-nothing exercise patterns with daily movement he genuinely enjoyed. He shifted from restrictive diet plans to gradual, permanent upgrades in food quality and eating patterns. He prioritized sleep as the foundation of health rather than a luxury to be sacrificed.

Most importantly, he extended his timeline. Rather than expecting transformation in weeks, he committed to a five-year vision of gradually improving health. This longer perspective allowed for sustainable changes, strategic patience, and the organic growth of new habits.

Three years into this approach, Alex achieved what had eluded him through decades of health warfare: lasting change. His weight stabilized at a healthy level without restriction. His formerly high blood pressure normalized without medication. His chronic joint pain resolved through consistent, appropriate movement. Most significantly, health practices that had once required willpower became automatic preferences.

Research supports this cultivation approach to long-term health. A study found that gradual lifestyle changes maintained for at least five years produced better health outcomes than more dramatic short-term interventions, even when the short-term approaches showed better immediate results.[7] Meanwhile, research demonstrates that habits integrated into natural life patterns show significantly higher long-term retention rates compared to behaviors perceived as separate from daily routines, which often have retention rates below 10% within a year.

Your long-term victory planning includes:

- Realistic timeline expectations based on biological realities
- Emphasis on systems over goals
- Strategic sequencing of health changes for maximum adherence
- Development of identity-based rather than compliance-based motivation
- Environmental design that makes healthy choices the default
- Social alignment that supports rather than undermines health vision

The wise general, Sun Tzu taught, wins the war before it begins. The wise health strategist similarly creates conditions where disease retreats not because it is defeated in battle, but because it can find no favorable terrain on which to advance.

The Campaign Begins: Your Strategic Health Plan

The general who attempts to implement all strategies simultaneously disperses forces and invites defeat. As you prepare to apply these principles, strategic prioritization is essential.

Begin with reconnaissance—a comprehensive assessment of your current health landscape across all five pillars. Identify your areas of strength and vulnerability without judgment. Like a general surveying territory, your goal is accuracy, not shame or pride.

Next, determine your highest leverage points—those areas where strategic intervention will create cascading benefits across multiple systems. For some, this might be sleep optimization, which improves hormonal regulation, inflammatory status, and cognitive function simultaneously. For others, it might be stress management, nutritional upgrades, or specific movement patterns.

Strategic Health Assessment Framework

"The general who wins a battle makes many calculations before the battle is fought."

Strategic Domain	Assessment Questions
Reconnaissance (Gathering with Intelligence)	• What health metrics have you measured in the past year? • What genetic predispositions run in your family? • What environmental factors most impact your health? • What early warning symptoms do you typically ignore?
Moral Law (Nutrition & Core Values)	• What core values guide your health decisions? • Do your food choices align with these values? • What nutritional approach makes you feel most vital? • What food traditions/background influence your choices?
Heaven (Environment & Biological Rhythms)	• How does your local climate affect your health? • When are your natural peak energy times? • What environmental toxins are you regularly exposed to? • How do seasonal changes affect your wellbeing?
Earth (Physical Body & Movement)	• What movement patterns feel most natural to you? • What physical limitations must you work around? • What activities give you joy rather than dread? • What physical strengths can you leverage?
Commander (Mental Resilience & Decision-making)	• How do you make decisions when temptation arises? • What thought patterns sabotage your health efforts? • How do you respond to setbacks and failures? • What mental health practices support your resilience?

"Know yourself, know your enemy. In a hundred battles, you will never be in peril."

Develop clear, measurable objectives for each phase of your campaign. Avoid the common mistake of vague aspirations ("get healthier") in favor of specific, observable outcomes ("reduce inflammatory markers," "improve sleep efficiency," "increase stress resilience").

Finally, remember Sun Tzu's emphasis on adaptability: "Just as water retains no constant shape, in warfare there are no constant conditions." Your health strategy must similarly evolve as your body changes, as science advances, and as life circumstances shift. The rigid general who cannot adapt to changing conditions will ultimately be defeated, regardless of initial advantages.

The art of health, like the art of war, is not a prescription but a process—a way of thinking strategically about the most precious territory you'll ever defend: your body. By applying Sun Tzu's wisdom to this intimate battlefield, you become not just a patient following orders but a general directing a campaign—observant, strategic, and ultimately victorious in the pursuit of lasting vitality.

Your body is the only home you'll never leave. Defend it wisely.

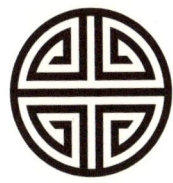

2

Mastering Health: The Economics of Wellness Maintenance

"Thus we may know that there are five essentials for victory: He will win who knows when to fight and when not to fight. He will win who knows how to handle both superior and inferior forces. He will win whose army is animated by the same spirit throughout all its ranks. He will win who, prepared himself, waits to take the enemy unprepared. He will win who has military capacity and is not interfered with by the sovereign." — Sun Tzu

The Besieged Fortress

Marcus sat in his kitchen, staring at the small mountain of pills before him: metformin for diabetes, lisinopril for hypertension, atorvastatin for cholesterol, and omeprazole for the acid reflux caused by the other medications. At 54, his medicine cabinet resembled a small pharmacy, costing him $437 each month—even with insurance.

Across town, Elena stretched on her yoga mat, moving through a sequence she'd practiced for years. At 62, she took no daily medications. Her kitchen cupboards housed herbs and spices rather than pharmaceuticals. Her annual medical expenses consisted mainly of preventive screenings and her monthly yoga studio membership.

Same city. Similar age. Dramatically different health economies.

When Sun Tzu wrote, "The art of war is of vital importance to the State. It is a matter of life and death, a road either to safety or to ruin," he could have been describing not just warfare but the intimate battles waged within our bodies. Your personal health economy—how you allocate resources, when you choose to deploy them, and which fronts you strengthen or neglect—determines whether you'll live in abundance or scarcity, freedom or constraint, vitality or deterioration.

Your body is a besieged fortress. The question is not whether attacks will come—they will, in forms ranging from viral invaders to inflammatory agents to oxidative stress. The question is: Will your defensive infrastructure be sound when they arrive? Will your soldiers be trained? Will your supply lines remain intact?

The Five Battlefronts of Health Economics

In Sun Tzu's framework, "He will win who knows when to fight and when not to fight." In health terms, this translates to strategic decision-making about where to allocate your precious resources.

Picture your health as defended on five interconnected fronts: the Treasury of Prevention (resources allocated before disease appears), the Arsenal of Early Intervention (resources deployed at the first sign of trouble), the Garrison of Chronic Management (resources committed to ongoing conditions), the Relief Corps of Acute Care (resources mobilized in emergencies), and the Intelligence Network of Monitoring (resources invested in surveillance and data).

Most modern health systems—and individuals—operate with a severely imbalanced strategy, pouring vast resources into the Relief Corps while leaving the Treasury nearly empty. We spend billions on emergency interventions but pennies on prevention. We deploy financial cavalry for heart attacks but balk at funding daily exercise. We marshal economic armies against stage 4 cancer but hesitate to provision healthy food systems.

This is not just financially unsound; it's strategically catastrophic.

Consider the evidence: For every $1 invested in childhood vaccines, society saves ~$16 in future healthcare costs. A $1 investment in workplace wellness programs returns approximately $3 in reduced healthcare spending. Each $1 allocated to smoking cessation programs saves ~$3 in treatment costs for tobacco-related diseases.[1]

These aren't merely statistics; they're battle plans. They reveal where the strategic health warrior should concentrate forces for maximum impact.

The Silent Siege: How Chronic Disease Drains Resources

When Sun Tzu wrote that "supreme excellence consists in breaking the enemy's resistance without fighting," he unwittingly described the ideal health strategy: prevent disease before it requires treatment.

The statistics tell a sobering story: chronic diseases consume 86% of all healthcare spending in America.[2] Each year, diabetes costs the average patient approximately $16,750 in medical expenses and lost productivity. Heart disease extracts ~$18,953 per patient. Cancer demands a staggering ~$42,000 per patient in direct medical costs alone.[3]

But these figures only account for visible costs. The invisible siege is equally devastating: the mental burden of managing multiple conditions, the energy diverted from creative pursuits to disease management, the narrowing of life's possibilities as health deteriorates, the strain on relationships as caregiving responsibilities increase, and the emotional toll of confronting mortality prematurely.

Consider Thomas, a 47-year-old architect who ignored early warning signs of hypertension. "I didn't have time for doctor visits," he explained. "I had deadlines, projects, a family depending on me." Ten years and one stroke later, his economic reality transformed: disability payments instead of a salary, a part-time caregiver, modifications to his home, and twenty-seven pills weekly. The cost of his "I don't have time" strategy? Approximately $1.3 million in lost income, healthcare expenses, and reduced quality of life.

The strategic health warrior recognizes this pattern and disrupts it before it begins.

The Economics of Swift Action

In battle, timing is everything. Sun Tzu observed that "rapidity is the essence of war," noting that elite forces strike with the speed of rolling thunder. In health, the same principle applies.

Consider breast cancer: Treatment at Stage 0 or 1 costs approximately $60,000 to $80,000, while treatment at Stage 4 ranges from ~$150,000 to $250,000.[4] This stark difference represents more than money; it represents suffering, disability, and mortality risk. Each day of delayed action increases all three.

Melissa, a 38-year-old teacher, noticed a small lump during a shower. Unlike many who might "wait and see," she acted immediately. "My mother died after finding a lump and waiting six months to see a doctor," she explained. "I called my doctor that same day." The mass, caught at Stage 1, required a lumpectomy and radiation but no chemotherapy. Total treatment cost: ~$67,500. Estimated cost had she waited until Stage 3: approximately $182,000, plus incalculable suffering.

The lesson is clear: in health as in warfare, swift action wins battles before they escalate into wars.

This principle applies equally to mental health. Research found that untreated depression costs approximately $10,000 annually per person in lost productivity and increased physical healthcare utilization. Early intervention with therapy ($500 to $2,000) yields a return on investment of 300 to 500%.

When Patricia, a marketing executive, recognized her anxiety was escalating beyond her control, she immediately sought therapy rather than "pushing through." Six sessions of cognitive-behavioral therapy (~$1,200) helped her develop effective management strategies. "My colleague had similar symptoms but self-medicated with alcohol for years," she noted. "She eventually needed inpatient treatment costing over ~$30,000, and she lost her job in the process."

Sun Tzu would approve of Patricia's strategy: decisive action at the first sign of vulnerability.

Strategic Allocation: The Five Terrains of Health Investment

The master strategist understands that not all investments yield equal returns. Sun Tzu identified five terrains on which battles are fought, each requiring different tactics. Similarly, health investments can be categorized by their strategic value:

1. The Disputed Ground: Reactive Medical Care

Most health spending occurs here—medications, procedures, hospitalizations. These are necessary but represent tactical retreats rather than strategic advances. They manage damage already done.

Consider statins, among the most commonly prescribed medications worldwide. At approximately $1,200 to $2,400 annually for brand-name versions (including monitoring), they reduce cardiovascular events by 25 to 30%. Effective, yes, but a reactive rather than proactive strategy.

2. The Accessible Ground: Basic Prevention

These low-barrier investments yield moderate returns: annual check-ups, standard screenings, basic supplements. Important, but insufficient alone.

Regular blood pressure monitoring costs approximately $30 to $100 for a home device, potentially preventing thousands in stroke-related expenses. A worthwhile investment, but still primarily focused on early detection rather than optimal function.

3. The Entangling Ground: Lifestyle Medicine

Here we find higher-impact investments that require more committed engagement: regular exercise, consistently healthy nutrition, stress management practices, quality sleep habits.

These require greater initial effort but yield compounding returns. Regular strength training, for instance, costs from nothing at all to about $100 monthly but reduces healthcare expenditures by approximately $2,500 annually for older adults through reduced falls, improved metabolic health, and maintained independence.

James, a 67-year-old retiree, invested in twice-weekly personal training sessions (~$400 monthly) after a pre-diabetes diagnosis. "My friends thought I was extravagant," he recalled. "But five years later, I'm on zero medications while they take handfuls. My 'extravagance' has saved me thousands annually in avoided medical costs."

4. The Open Ground: Environmental Optimization

These investments focus on creating surroundings that naturally support health: high-quality water filtration, air purification, non-toxic household products, ergonomic workspaces.

The returns here are difficult to quantify precisely but potentially enormous. Consider that removing endocrine-disrupting chemicals from your environment may reduce cancer risk, improve fertility, and enhance metabolic function—all without ongoing effort once the initial changes are made.

Maya, an accountant with recurring migraines, spent ~$3,800 updating her home's water filtration system, replacing synthetic bedding with natural materials, and installing air purifiers. "My neurologist thought I was wasting money," she said. "But my migraines decreased by 80% within three months. I went from missing work monthly to missing almost none, and I've been able to discontinue three medications."

5. The Key Ground: Mindset and Knowledge

The highest-leverage investments occur here: health education, medical literacy, self-assessment skills, and psychological frameworks for decision-making.

These investments transform every other health expenditure by ensuring resources flow to high-value targets. They're the ultimate asymmetric warfare in health—small inputs creating massive outputs.

When Richard, a 59-year-old sales manager, spent ~$1,200 on a specialized health education program, his colleagues were skeptical. Three years later, he had reduced his annual healthcare costs by approximately $8,700 through improved medical decision-making, avoidance of unnecessary procedures, and prevention strategies tailored to his genetic profile.

"Understanding my body's workings and the healthcare system's incentives gave me a strategic advantage," he explained. "I now make decisions like a general deploying troops, not a casualty awaiting rescue."

The Invisible Advantage: Compound Returns on Health Investments

Sun Tzu wrote, "To secure ourselves against defeat lies in our own hands, but the opportunity of defeating the enemy is provided by the enemy himself." In health terms, this means your daily choices determine your vulnerability, while disease reveals itself through early warning signs—if you're trained to recognize them.

Most health investments compound, creating returns far exceeding their initial cost. Consider three examples:

The 10,000-Step Strategy
Walking 10,000 steps daily costs little more than time. Over ten years, this habit can lead to significant benefits: approximately $7,200 saved in direct medical costs, $16,000 in avoided productivity losses, and two to four additonal quality life years, valued at roughly $200,000 to $400,000. Combined, the total 10-year return could range from $223,200 to $423,200, with no monetary investment required.[5]

The Mediterranean Meal Plan

Adhering to a Mediterranean diet may cost approximately $2 to $4 more daily than a standard American diet (~$730 to $1,460 annually). Over twenty years, this investment can yield significant returns: approximately $18,000 saved in direct cardiovascular disease expenses, $12,000 saved in diabetes-related costs, $23,000 saved in cancer-related expenses, and three to five additional quality life years, valued at roughly $300,000 to $500,000. Combined, the total 20-year return could range from $353,000 to $553,000 on a ~$14,600 to $29,200 investment.[6]

The Sleep Restoration Project

Investing ~$1,500 in sleep optimization (quality mattress, blackout curtains, sleep tracking) can yield significant returns: approximately $3,800 annually in improved productivity, $2,200 annually in reduced healthcare utilization, and a reduction in dementia risk valued at roughly $5,000 to $10,000 annually (based on future care costs). Over ten years, the total return could range from $110,000 to $160,000 on a ~$1,500 investment.[7]

These calculations exclude the incalculable: the joy of pain-free movement, the pleasure of sustained cognitive function, the freedom of independence in later years. These are the true dividends of strategic health investment.

The Fallacy of Deferred Maintenance

"There is no instance of a country having benefited from prolonged warfare," wrote Sun Tzu. Similarly, there is no instance of a body benefiting from prolonged neglect.

Modern healthcare systems often operate on a deferred maintenance model: ignore small problems until they become catastrophes. This approach makes as much sense as ignoring small leaks in a roof until the ceiling collapses.

Consider diabetes, which progresses through identifiable stages: insulin resistance (reversible through lifestyle, cost: ~$0 to $500 annually), prediabetes (reversible through more intensive lifestyle intervention, cost: ~$500 to $2,000 annually), early diabetes (potentially reversible, management cost: ~$2,000 to $5,000 annually), and advanced diabetes with complications (irreversible, management cost: ~$10,000 to $20,000+ annually).[8] Each year of deferred maintenance increases lifetime costs exponentially.

Rebecca, a human resources director, discovered her blood glucose was trending upward at age 42. Rather than waiting for a diabetes diagnosis, she immediately implemented a metabolic health program. "It cost me ~$3,200 that year between a continuous glucose monitor, a health coach, and a gym membership," she recalled. "Five years later, my glucose is normal, and I've avoided medication entirely."

Her colleague Michael, with similar blood glucose levels, decided to "wait and see." Five years later, he manages diabetes with multiple medications costing approximately $4,800 annually, with projections suggesting his lifetime diabetes-related expenses will exceed ~$300,000.

The strategic health warrior recognizes that maintenance is infinitely cheaper than repair, both financially and biologicaly.

The Competitive Advantage of Health

In Sun Tzu's world, victory went to armies with superior strategy, morale, and leadership. In the modern world, similar advantages accrue to those with superior health.

The evidence is striking: Workers with higher well-being are about 13% more productive; employees who eat healthy all day are 25% more likely to have higher job performance (and have ~27% lower absenteeism); executives who exercise regularly are rated higher on leadership effectiveness; and students with healthier diets and regular breakfast tend to perform better academically.[9] These findings highlight a fundamental truth: health is far more than the absence of disease—it is a strategic advantage that enhances performance and success in every domain of life.

When Sarah, a corporate attorney, invested two hours daily in health practices—morning exercise, meditation, meal preparation, and early bedtime—colleagues questioned her priorities. "They'd work until midnight while I left at 6 PM," she recalled. "But over time, my clear thinking and sustained energy became apparent. I began outperforming colleagues who worked longer hours but neglected their health. Eventually, my approach became a competitive advantage—my health investments yielded professional returns."

Sun Tzu would recognize Sarah's strategy as the epitome of asymmetric warfare: modest investments generating outsized returns.

The Health Sovereign's Dilemma

Sun Tzu wrote, "The general who wins a battle makes many calculations in his temple before the battle is fought." Similarly, the health sovereign—you—must make critical calculations before deploying resources.

Every health decision involves tradeoffs between immediate vs. delayed benefits, visible vs. invisible returns, effort vs. outcome, and individual vs. collective action. These calculations aren't merely financial; they're philosophical. They reveal your values, time preference, and risk tolerance.

Consider three individuals facing identical hypertension

diagnoses:

> **Carlos, the Minimalist:** "I'll take the prescribed medication (~$360 annually), continue my current lifestyle, and accept the statistical outcomes." Time investment: minimal. Financial investment: moderate. Projected outcome: managed disease with gradual progression.
>
> **Ling, the Optimizer:** "I'll implement lifestyle changes (Mediterranean diet, stress reduction, exercise) while using medication temporarily." Time investment: significant. Financial investment: moderate. Projected outcome: potential medication elimination and disease reversal.
>
> **David, the Maximalist:** "I'll overhaul my environment and lifestyle completely, seek specialized testing to identify root causes, and use targeted supplementation alongside conventional care." Time investment: extensive. Financial investment: substantial. Projected outcome: comprehensive health optimization beyond single disease management.

None of these approaches is inherently right or wrong—each represents a strategic choice with associated benefits and costs. The wise health sovereign chooses consciously rather than defaulting to the path of least resistance.

The Ultimate Victory: Health Sovereignty

Sun Tzu's ultimate teaching is that the greatest victory requires no battle. Applied to health, this means creating conditions where disease cannot take hold—not through constant warfare against symptoms, but through strategic prevention and health optimization.

This approach requires a shift in thinking from reactive to proactive, from fragmented to integrated, from disease-focused to vitality-focused, and from passive to sovereign.

Health sovereignty means recognizing yourself as the primary decision-maker, resource-allocator, and strategist in your health campaign. It means understanding that while healthcare providers are important allies, the ultimate responsibility for your health strategy rests with you.

When Nicole, a teacher diagnosed with an autoimmune condition, was told she would require lifelong medications, she accepted the prescription but didn't accept the prognosis. "I became the general of my own health campaign," she explained. "I researched extensively, assembled a diverse team of health allies, eliminated inflammatory triggers from my environment, adopted meditation for stress management, and completely redesigned my nutrition. Five years later, my markers were normal, and my rheumatologist now uses my case as a teaching example."

This isn't magical thinking—it's strategy. Nicole applied Sun Tzu's principle of knowing herself (her genetic predis-

Strategic Health Investment: Comparative ROI

"In battle, there are not more than two methods of attack: the direct and the indirect." —Sun Tzu

Investment Category	Initial Cost	10-Year Return	Strategic Value
Reactive Medical (medications, procedures)	$$$ $2,000–$20,000/year	10–30% Symptom management	●○○○○
Basic Prevention (screenings, checkups)	$$ $500–$2,000/year	50–100% Early detection	●●○○○
Lifestyle Medicine (exercise, nutrition, sleep)	$$ $1,000–$5,000/year	200–500% Disease prevention	●●●●○
Environmental Optimization (water, air, living space)	$$$ $2,000–10,000 initial	300–700% Toxin reduction	●●●●○
Mindset and Knowledge (education, medical literacy)	$ $500–$2,000 initial	500–1000% Decision optimization	●●●●●

positions, specific inflammatory triggers, unique responses to interventions) and knowing her enemy (the mechanisms, patterns, and vulnerabilities of her condition). Armed with this knowledge, she fought not with desperation but with precision.

The Warrior's Health Economy: A New Paradigm

Sun Tzu taught that "the wise warrior avoids the battle." Similarly, the wise health sovereign avoids the hospital—not through fear or neglect, but through strategic prevention.

This requires a new economic paradigm: Invest Upstream by allocating resources to prevention and early intervention; Value the Invisible by recognizing that the absence of disease represents a return on investment; Calculate Lifetime Value by considering the long-term returns of health decisions; Diversify Health Assets by building physical, mental, and social health capital simultaneously; and Maintain Strategic Reserves by preserving energy, vitality, and resources for unexpected health challenges.

Those who adopt this paradigm create a fundamentally different health economy—one characterized by abundance rather than scarcity, freedom rather than constraint, and sovereignty rather than dependence.

When Elena, now 62 and medication-free, passes Marcus at the pharmacy counter, both are living the consequences of distinct health economies. Elena's daily yoga, whole-food nutrition, meaningful social connections, and environmental optimizations represent investments that have compounded over decades. Marcus's regimen of pills represents the accumulated interest on health debt—payments that manage but rarely eliminate the underlying liability.

The difference between their health economies wasn't income, access, or luck. It was strategy—specifically, what

Sun Tzu might call the economics of prevention versus the economics of reaction.

The choice between these economies is yours to make, not once but daily. Each meal, movement, thought pattern, and environmental exposure represents an economic transaction in your personal health marketplace. Each strengthens either the forces of vitality or the forces of dysfunction.

The art of mastering health, like the art of war, lies not in dramatic interventions but in consistent strategy—the accumulated advantage of thousands of small, wise choices that ultimately determine not just how long you live, but how well you live.

Choose wisely, health warrior. Your campaign has already begun.

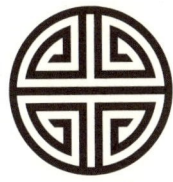

3

Attack by Stratagem: Winning with Preventive Measures

"Unless it is absolutely necessary, never use force when taking control of another state." — Sun Tzu

The Silent Battlefield Where Most Victories Go Uncelebrated

Imagine your body as a kingdom under constant threat of invasion. Not from marauding armies with banners and trumpets announcing their arrival, but from silent infiltrators—pathogens slipping past border guards, cellular rebels orchestrating coups from within, microscopic saboteurs corrupting your metabolic supply chains.

In this strange war, the most spectacular victories are the ones that make no headlines. They are the cancers that never form, the heart attacks that never strike, the autoimmune rebellions that never materialize.

Richard never understood this paradox until it was too late.

He sat in his oncologist's office, a 52-year-old financial analyst who had spent decades mastering probability and risk in markets but had somehow failed to apply those same principles to his own body. Stage 3 colon cancer. The enemy had established territory, built fortifications, and was threatening to expand its occupation.

"If only we had caught this earlier," his doctor said, reviewing the neglected follow-up appointment from two years prior. "The polyp they found during your colonoscopy—the one you postponed removing—that's where this began."

Richard had prioritized quarterly earnings reports over quarterly health check-ins. Now, instead of a simple outpatient procedure that would have required a single afternoon, he faced chemotherapy, radiation, surgery—the full-scale invasion of his own body by medical necessity.

What would Sun Tzu say about such a strategic failure?

Perhaps this: *"The skillful leader subdues the enemy's troops without any fighting; he captures their cities without laying siege to them; he overthrows their kingdom without lengthy operations in the field."*

The Unorthodox Mathematics of Prevention: Zero as the Ultimate Victory

In the standard medical paradigm, success is measured by survival rates, remission statistics, and recovery timelines. This inverted logic celebrates the victory of returning to baseline after crisis rather than avoiding crisis altogether.

A prominent neuroscientist captures this paradox perfectly: "We value the dramatic rescue over the maintenance of health. We'd rather fall off a cliff and be heroically rescued than simply avoid the cliff in the first place."

Consider these mathematical realities: The conventional healthcare equation celebrates when 90% of heart attack victims survive. The preventive healthcare equation celebrates when those heart attacks never occur at all—a reduction of up to 80% through optimal lifestyle interventions.

Research estimates that 30 to 50% of all cancers are preventable through lifestyle factors.[1] Yet our medical system invests billions in treatment while allocating mere pennies to teaching these preventive strategies. Research from major diabetes prevention initiatives shows that up to 58% of type 2 diabetes cases are preventable through targeted lifestyle interventions, yet the CDC reports that more than 80% of prediabetic Americans remain unaware of their condition.[2]

Which victory is more complete—surviving disease or preventing it entirely?

The Tale of Two Brothers: A Zero-Sum Game Where Zero Wins

David and Michael Rodriguez shared the same genetic inheritance—a father dead at 47 from a massive coronary, a mother battling type 2 diabetes, grandparents claimed by various cardiovascular calamities. Their genetic dice were loaded with metabolic time bombs.

But they played those dice differently.

David, believing destiny was fixed, lived reactively. When his blood pressure rose at 42, he grudgingly took medication. When his cholesterol followed at 45, he added another pill. At 52, chest pain sent him to the emergency room—a 95% blockage in his left anterior descending artery, requiring emergency stenting. The procedure cost approximately $38,000. The subsequent cardiac rehabilitation program added approximately $8,600. Lifetime medication costs: approximately $4,000 annually. The invisible costs—reduced stamina, psychological uncertainty, career limitations—remain incalculable.

Michael approached his genetic inheritance as Sun Tzu might approach an enemy with known tendencies and predictable tactics. At 35, he underwent comprehensive cardiovascular assessment, identifying early signs of the same vulnerabilities that would later ambush his brother. Instead of waiting for symptoms, he deployed a multi-faceted preventive strategy.

He adopted nutrition optimized for cardiovascular health, emphasizing the components of the Mediterranean diet proven to reduce heart disease risk by 30%. He implemented a strategic exercise regimen targeting both cardiorespiratory fitness and muscle mass, reducing cardiovascular mortality risk by up to 50%. He practiced stress management reducing inflammation markers by 15 to 20% and prioritized sleep optimization, reducing heart disease risk by 34%.

Total annual cost: approximately $3,500 in preventive care, specialized testing, and quality food.

At 57, Michael's cardiovascular age tests 15 years younger than his chronological age. No medications. No procedures. No emergencies.

David survived his heart attack. Conventional medicine would count this as a success.

Michael never had a heart attack to survive. Preventive strategy would count this as the greater victory.

As Sun Tzu observed: "To win one hundred victories in one hundred battles is not the acme of skill. To subdue the enemy without fighting is the acme of skill."

The Five Battlegrounds of Health:
Unconventional Warfare on Conventional Disease

Sun Tzu identified five methods of attack, arranged in order of preference. These translate to health with surprising precision, though not in ways your doctor is likely to discuss during your 15-minute appointment.

1. Disrupt the Enemy's Plans Before They Materialize

The highest form of prevention occurs when disease cannot even organize its forces.

When Amara discovered she carried the BRCA1 gene mutation at age 32, increasing her lifetime breast cancer risk to 72%,[3] she faced a crossroads. Conventional wisdom offered mammograms starting at 25, MRIs, and the eventual probability of prophylactic surgery.

Instead, Amara deployed a strategy that made her body hostile territory for cancer development. She optimized estrogen metabolism through targeted nutrition and specific cruciferous compound supplementation, shown to favorably modify estrogen breakdown pathways. She implemented intermittent fasting protocols demonstrated to reduce cancer incidence by 35% in high-risk populations and maintained a regular exercise regimen proven to increase natural killer cell activity by up to 60%.

She minimized exposure to xenoestrogens and endocrine disruptors while optimizing vitamin D levels—associated with 50% lower breast cancer incidence in BRCA carriers maintaining levels above 60 ng/mL.

Ten years later, at 42, Amara remains cancer-free, with breast tissue density and inflammatory markers that continue to improve rather than worsen with age.

This approach doesn't guarantee she'll never develop cancer. But she's systematically undermining cancer's ability to establish itself—disrupting its supply lines, communication systems, and growth environment before it can even organize its attack.

2. Disrupt Alliances: The Unusual Suspects in Disease Confederacies

Disease rarely operates alone. It forms alliances—unholy confederacies of compounding factors that amplify each other's effects.

Consider the metabolic alliance known as "The Deadly Quartet": insulin resistance, hypertension, dyslipidemia, and visceral adiposity. When these four allies coordinate their attack, the risk of cardiovascular events increases significantly. Yet conventional medicine often treats each as an isolated condition with a separate medication.

Robert, a 45-year-old software engineer with prediabetes, hypertension, and elevated triglycerides, was prescribed three medications by three different specialists. None discussed how these conditions were interconnected. None addressed the shared root causes.

Following Sun Tzu's principle of disrupting enemy alliances, Robert researched the common pathways underlying all three conditions. He discovered the connecting thread—chronic inflammation and insulin dysregulation—and developed a counterinsurgency strategy.

He adopted time-restricted eating patterns shown to improve insulin sensitivity by 58% within 12 weeks. He implemented Zone 2 cardiovascular training combined with resistance exercise, demonstrated to reduce inflammatory cytokines by 30 to 40%. He eliminated pro-inflammatory foods identified through advanced testing and strategically incorporated polyphenol-rich foods proven to modulate

NF-κB inflammatory pathways.

Six months later, Robert's metabolic alliance had collapsed—blood pressure normalized, blood glucose stabilized, triglycerides reduced by 62%. His doctor, both impressed and slightly defensive, suggested he might "reduce some of his medications."

3. Attack the Army: When Direct Engagement Becomes Necessary

Sometimes, even the most vigilant strategist must face an enemy directly. When prevention fails or wasn't implemented in time, direct confrontation becomes necessary.

For Sophia, diagnosed with HER2-positive breast cancer at 41, this meant surgery, chemotherapy, and targeted biological therapy. But even in direct battle, Sun Tzu's principles remained relevant: "If you know the enemy and know yourself, you need not fear the result of a hundred battles."

Working with an integrative oncologist, Sophia deployed conventional treatments while simultaneously implementing fasting protocols shown to reduce chemotherapy side effects by up to 40% and improve effectiveness.[5] She utilized specific exercise interventions demonstrated to improve chemotherapy completion rates by 30% and employed evidence-based complementary approaches to target cancer's specific metabolic vulnerabilities. She addressed sleep disruption, shown to reduce cancer recurrence risk by 50%.

Sophia's oncologist initially dismissed these approaches as irrelevant. Three months later, when her tumor response exceeded expectations and her side effects remained minimal, the same oncologist began asking questions about her complementary protocol.

According to multiple integrative medicine research institutions, patients combining conventional treatment with evidence-based complementary approaches report 35 to 50% better quality of life, 25 to 30% fewer side effects, and may experience improved treatment outcomes in certain cancer types.

4. Attack Cities: The Siege Warfare of Last Resort

"The worst policy is to attack cities," Sun Tzu cautioned. In health terms, this represents the most invasive interventions—emergency surgeries, intensive care, transplants, and other heroic measures that, while sometimes necessary, extract tremendous costs.

James ignored escalating symptoms of type 2 diabetes for years, declining preventive strategies and rejecting lifestyle modifications. "When something serious happens, they'll fix it," he told his concerned wife.

At 57, that "something serious" arrived—a massive stroke followed by kidney failure, requiring ICU admission, dialysis, and extensive rehabilitation. The financial cost exceeded approximately $350,000 in the first year alone. The human cost included permanent disability, dependency, and dramatically reduced quality of life.

Research reports that approximately 70% of healthcare spending in the United States goes toward treating preventable chronic conditions. Meanwhile, only 2.9% of healthcare dollars are invested in prevention. This inverted resource allocation reflects a system designed to besiege cities rather than outmaneuver enemies before walls become necessary.

5. Defense as a Last Resort: The Holding Pattern of Symptom Management

"Invincibility lies in the defense; the possibility of victory in the attack." Sun Tzu recognized that while defensive postures are sometimes necessary, they rarely lead to victory.

Elena's experience with chronic migraines illustrates this

principle perfectly. For seven years, she relied on increasingly powerful pain medications to manage attacks that came with greater frequency and intensity. Each new drug worked briefly before losing effectiveness, requiring higher doses or different compounds. This defensive strategy kept her functioning but offered no path to victory.

The turning point came when a neurologist trained in functional medicine suggested they stop defending against attacks and instead launch a coordinated offensive against the root causes. Advanced testing revealed several interconnected factors: undiagnosed non-celiac gluten sensitivity (associated with a 400% increased risk of migraine[6]), estrogen dominance exacerbating neuroinflammation during specific cycle phases, magnesium deficiency affecting neuronal excitability, sleep-disrupted breathing causing nocturnal hypoxia, and dysfunctional cervical biomechanics creating vascular compression.

Addressing these root factors reduced Elena's migraine frequency by 92% within three months. After a year, she experienced complete resolution—a true victory rather than an endless defensive battle.

Leading headache research organizations note that while 39 million Americans suffer from migraines, fewer than 12% receive comprehensive care addressing underlying causes. Most remain trapped in defensive symptom management that promises survival but never victory.

The Unconventional Alliance: Reimagining the Doctor-Patient Relationship

"The wise general thinks of victory in terms of alliances." Sun Tzu understood that no leader, however brilliant, succeeds alone. In health terms, your most powerful alliance is with

healthcare providers—but perhaps not in the way you've been taught to think about this relationship.

The conventional medical model positions the doctor as general and the patient as foot soldier—expected to follow orders without question. A strategic health alliance inverts this hierarchy.

Thomas, diagnosed with early-stage prostate cancer at 64, was immediately scheduled for radical prostatectomy. When he requested time to research options, his urologist warned that delay could be deadly. Unsatisfied with this pressure, Thomas sought a more strategic partnership.

He assembled a team including a urologist specializing in active surveillance, an integrative oncologist, a nutritional therapist specializing in cancer metabolism, and a mind-body specialist. Together, they developed a comprehensive approach combining active surveillance with regular PSA testing and advanced imaging, a nutritional protocol focusing on compounds shown to specifically target prostate cancer cells, a targeted exercise regimen demonstrated to slow prostate cancer progression by 57%, and stress management practices proven to normalize cortisol patterns associated with slower cancer growth.

Five years later, Thomas's cancer remains indolent—unchanged in volume or aggression. The statistics support his approach: According to major prostate cancer research centers, up to 60% of prostate cancers diagnosed today are non-aggressive and may never require surgical intervention, yet most men still undergo immediate radical treatment with significant quality-of-life impacts.

The strategic health warrior recognizes that modern medicine excels at certain types of battles—acute interventions, emergency care, advanced diagnostics—while often struggling with others—prevention, lifestyle optimization, addressing root causes of chronic conditions. The wisest strategy involves recruiting the right allies for each specific health challenge rather than expecting any single approach to win all battles.

Intelligence Gathering: The Unspoken Foundation of Prevention

"What enables the wise sovereign and the good general to strike and conquer, and achieve things beyond the reach of ordinary men, is foreknowledge." For Sun Tzu, intelligence was the foundation of strategy.

In health terms, this means regular, strategic assessment of your current status, risk factors, and early warning signs—not just the basic screening recommended for the general population.

Consider these disquieting statistics: Standard cholesterol panels miss 50% of people at risk for heart attacks.[7] Traditional diabetes screening fails to identify insulin resistance until pancreatic function has declined by over 60% according to endocrinology research. Conventional cancer screening often detects disease only after it has been developing for years or decades.

When Elena learned that her grandmother, mother, and aunt had all developed severe osteoporosis leading to life-altering fractures, she recognized a pattern that demanded advanced intelligence gathering.

Rather than waiting for the standard DEXA scan recommended for women at 65, she pursued comprehensive bone health assessment in her late thirties. She obtained specialized bone turnover markers showing the dynamic process of bone formation and resorption, comprehensive nutrient testing beyond standard calcium, inflammatory markers affecting osteoclast activity, hormonal panels assessing factors influencing bone metabolism, and genetic testing for variants affecting vitamin D utilization and collagen formation.

These tests revealed early signs of accelerated bone loss two decades before conventional screening would have caught the problem. Armed with this intelligence, Elena implemented a science-based protocol with weight-bearing exercise specifically designed to increase bone mineral density, shown to improve bone formation by up to 22%, targeted nutritional intervention with nutrients demonstrated to improve bone microarchitecture, hormone optimization appropriate for her age and specific needs, and strategic supplementation based on her genetic vulnerabilities.

Ten years later, at 47, Elena's bone density exceeds the average for her age group despite her strong genetic predisposition to osteoporosis. Research showed that this proactive approach reduces lifetime fracture risk by 30 to 70% when started before significant bone loss occurs.

The strategic health warrior recognizes that standardized screening schedules designed for population management often fail the individual. True intelligence gathering must be personalized to your specific risks, health history, genetics, and health objectives.

The Five Terrain Factors: Your Health Battleground Reimagined

Sun Tzu identified five factors that determine military success: moral influence, weather, terrain, command, and doctrine. These translate to health strategy with unexpected precision.

Moral Influence (Purpose and Values)
Why do you seek health? The most powerful motivation

comes not from fear of disease but from alignment with deeper purpose.

William initially approached health habits as bitter medicine—exercises he hated, foods he didn't enjoy, medical appointments he dreaded. Unsurprisingly, his adherence was poor. The transformation came when he connected his health to his core purpose—being present for his grandchildren's lives, having the vitality to teach them fishing and hiking as his grandfather had taught him.

Research from long-term studies of human happiness confirms that purpose-driven health behaviors persist at rates 300% higher than those motivated by fear or obligation.

Weather (Timing and Seasons)

Just as generals must adapt to changing weather conditions, health warriors must recognize the seasons of life and timing of interventions.

The interventions appropriate at 30 differ from those at 60. The strategy useful during career-building years may require modification during retirement. The approach beneficial during stress may need adjustment during grief.

When Liza applied the same high-intensity exercise regimen she'd used successfully in her thirties to her perimenopausal body at 48, she experienced worsening insomnia, increased inflammation, and accelerated weight gain. Her hormonal weather had changed, requiring a shift to strategically timed strength training and zone 2 cardio that reduced cortisol impact while maintaining muscle mass.

Terrain (Your Unique Biology)

Your genetic makeup, microbiome, medical history, and living environment collectively form your health terrain. A strategy that succeeds on one terrain may fail spectacularly on another.

When Susan followed the Mediterranean diet widely praised for cardiovascular health, she experienced worsening autoimmune symptoms and weight gain. Comprehensive testing revealed specific genetic variants affecting her response to certain fats, histamine intolerance exacerbated by fermented Mediterranean staples, and gut dysbiosis creating adverse reactions to foods considered universally "healthy."

A personalized protocol addressing her specific terrain produced results within weeks, while the "evidence-based" approach for the average person had caused deterioration.

Research recognizes that genetic variations affect how individuals respond to everything from caffeine to exercise to medication, with differences in effectiveness ranging from 30 to 300% based on specific polymorphisms.

Command (Personal Agency and Healthcare Relationships)
Who makes decisions about your health? The most successful outcomes occur when you maintain strategic command while tactically delegating specific tasks to appropriate specialists.

After a misdiagnosis nearly led to unnecessary surgery, Marcus redesigned his approach to healthcare interactions. He arrived at appointments with organized health data, specific questions, and a clear understanding of his options. He respectfully discussed alternatives, asked for evidence supporting recommendations, and made collaborative but independent decisions.

This approach initially surprised his providers, but ultimately earned their respect. His outcomes improved dramatically.

Research finds that patients who actively participate in medical decision-making experience 31% better treatment adherence, 26% higher satisfaction, and often superior clinical outcomes.[8]

Doctrine (Evidence-Based Principles)

Amid constantly shifting health trends, certain principles remain consistently supported by evidence. These form the doctrine of effective health strategy, though their specific application must be adapted to individual circumstances.

Research identifies several universal health determinants that transcend individual variation: whole food nutrition emphasizing plants, regular physical activity, adequate sleep, stress management, social connection, environmental health, and minimization of toxin exposure.

These fundamental doctrines provide strategic direction while allowing tactical flexibility based on individual needs.

The Invisible Victory: Celebrating What Never Happens

We return to the paradox that opened this chapter: in preventive health, the greatest victories are the events that never occur.

When Marcus implemented his comprehensive cardiovascular strategy and subsequently didn't have a heart attack, there was no dramatic victory to celebrate—no heroic surgery, no inspiring survival story, no "before and after" transformation. Just a healthy 65-year-old enjoying his grandchildren with an energy that seems unremarkable until compared with his chronological peers.

This invisibility of success represents both the challenge and the opportunity of preventive health. The challenge lies in maintaining motivation for actions whose benefits manifest primarily as non-events. The opportunity lies in redefining victory itself—from the dramatic rescue to the journey never requiring rescue.

As the ancient strategist might observe: "The supreme art of health is to prevent disease without fighting it."

The Strategic Health Manifesto

As you develop your own health stratagem, consider these principles drawn from Sun Tzu's wisdom:

Know yourself and your enemy. Understand your specific risk factors, genetic predispositions, and the particular diseases most likely to threaten your well-being.

Invest in intelligence. Regularly gather information about your health status through appropriate screenings, assessments, and self-monitoring.

Focus resources where they matter most. Direct your preventive efforts toward your highest-probability threats rather than dispersing energy across unlikely scenarios.

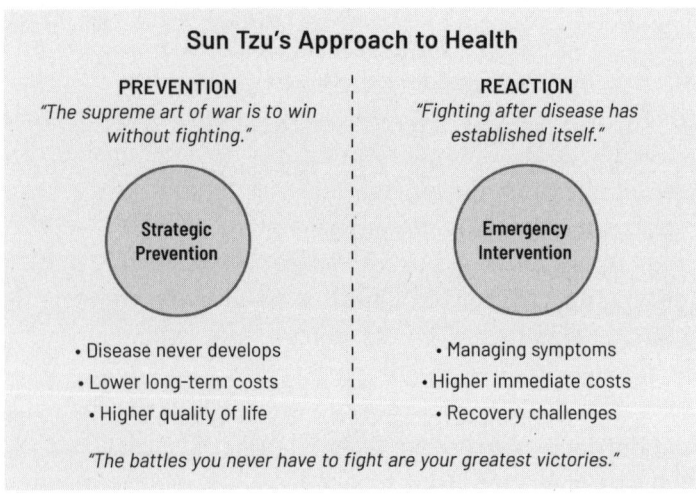

Build strategic alliances. Develop relationships with healthcare providers who respect your role as the commander of your health while offering valuable expertise.

Prepare the terrain. Create conditions in your body and environment that naturally resist disease rather than invite it.

ATTACK BY STRATAGEM: WINNING WITH PREVENTIVE MEASURES

Maintain flexibility. Adapt your strategy as circumstances change, new evidence emerges, and your body evolves.

Remember the ultimate goal. The purpose of health is not merely the absence of disease but the presence of vitality that enables you to fully engage with life's purpose.

Celebrate the invisible victories. Take time to acknowledge the diseases you've prevented, the crises averted, the quality of life preserved through strategic foresight.

In Sun Tzu's ancient wisdom lies a revolutionary truth for modern health: the battles you never have to fight represent your greatest triumphs. The health warrior's true art lies not in dramatic intervention but in the daily discipline of prevention—the quiet, consistent actions that collectively create a life of vibrant well-being, capable of fulfilling your highest purpose without the burden of preventable disease.

The wisest general sees farther, plans better, and acts earlier than his adversary. The wisest health strategist does the same.

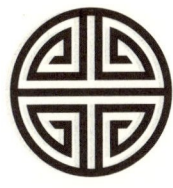

4

Tactical Dispositions: Positioning Yourself for Health Success

"The good fighters of old first put themselves beyond the possibility of defeat, and then waited for an opportunity to defeat the enemy." — Sun Tzu

The Invisible Fortress

Perhaps the most profound paradox in Sun Tzu's military wisdom comes when he speaks of invincibility: "One may know how to conquer without being able to do it." In health, as in warfare, the master tactician doesn't achieve victory through dramatic interventions but through positioning so impeccable that battles rarely materialize. The art isn't in healing sickness, but in creating conditions where sickness struggles to find purchase.

Consider the revelation that stunned public health officials during the 2009 H1N1 pandemic: why did some exposed individuals never contract the virus despite identical exposure conditions? Their immune positioning—shaped by sleep quality, prior exposures, microbiome composition, and stress chemistry—created what researchers now call "effective immunity" even without specific antibodies. Position, not intervention, determined their outcomes.[1]

The Harvard's landmark Nurses' Health Study revealed something equally counterintuitive: 82% of heart attacks among women could be prevented not through medications or procedures but through the invisible fortress created by five positional factors: nutrition, physical activity, body weight, smoking abstention, and moderate alcohol consumption.[2] The positioning fundamentally altered the terrain where disease sought to establish itself.

This unseen fortress—this tactical positioning—represents health's deepest truth: your body isn't a battlefield where you wage war against disease, but a kingdom whose defenses you either strengthen or compromise with every choice.

The Tactical Paradox

"To ensure that your whole host may withstand the brunt of the enemy's attack and remain unshaken—this is effected by maneuvers direct and indirect."

Marcus seemed to have health figured out. A marathoner with textbook vital signs and immaculate bloodwork, he positioned himself in what appeared to be perfect defensive formation. Yet at 42, during a routine screening, he received devastating news: Stage 3 colon cancer. How could someone so apparently "healthy" harbor such severe disease?

The paradox reveals a profound truth about health positioning: visible metrics often mask invisible vulnerabilities. Marcus had optimized cardiovascular fitness while neglecting cellular resilience. His low-fiber, high-protein diet, coupled with chronic sleep restriction and unprocessed emotional trauma, created what oncologists call "the perfect storm of cellular distress signaling." His positioning appeared robust from one perspective while harboring catastrophic vulnerability from another.

This illustrates what the Mayo Clinic's Dr. Michael Joyner calls "the measurement trap"—overvaluing what we can easily measure (blood pressure, cholesterol, weight) while undervaluing what we cannot (cellular stress response, mitochondrial function, nervous system regulation). The master health tactician recognizes that true positioning encompasses both visible and invisible domains.

The sobering statistics reveal this tactical paradox in population terms: Despite spending approximately $4.3 trillion annually on healthcare—more than any other nation—the U.S. ranks among the lower tier of developed countries in life expectancy.[3] We've positioned ourselves to excel at treating established disease while remaining vulnerable to its development. We've mastered offensive capability while neglecting defensive positioning.

The Four Positions of Health Mastery

"The skillful warrior first makes himself invulnerable, and then watches for vulnerability in his opponents."

Ancient Chinese medicine recognized four tactical positions in health maintenance that mirror Sun Tzu's military wisdom. Each represents a distinct relationship between the body and potential disease:

1. The Position of Prevention (上善若水—"Supreme good is like water")

Elisa, a 38-year-old architect, exemplifies this position. Despite a family history dense with cardiovascular disease, her inflammatory markers remain pristine. Her tactical positioning didn't emerge from heroic interventions but from the water-like quality of her daily choices—flowing naturally toward health-supporting behaviors not through willpower but through environmental design.

Her office features a standing desk positioned near natural light. Her home sits within walking distance of daily necessities. Her social circle engages primarily in active recreation. Her kitchen contains no ultra-processed foods because she never purchases them. Her bedtime arrives consistently because her evening routine makes sleep the path of least resistance.

This positioning aligns with the finding that 80% of premature heart disease, stroke, and type 2 diabetes—and 40% of cancers—could be prevented through lifestyle positioning rather than medical intervention. The position of prevention doesn't fight disease; it creates conditions where disease struggles to establish itself.[4]

2. The Position of Early Detection (知己知彼—"Know yourself, know your enemy")

"If you know the enemy and know yourself, your victory will not stand in doubt."

Maria, age 45, positions herself neither in paranoia nor neglect but in tactical surveillance. Unlike peers who avoid health information out of fear or those who compulsively seek diagnoses, Maria established what oncologists call "personalized health intelligence gathering."

She knows her specific genetic vulnerabilities through testing. She tracks inflammatory markers contextually against her behaviors. She conducts regular preventive screenings based on her personal risk profile rather than generic guidelines. When minor symptoms appear, she neither ignores them nor catastrophizes, but investigates their patterns within her body's unique language.

This position aligns with the finding that early-stage cancers have survival rates approaching 90%, while late-stage diagnoses drop below 20%. It mirrors the CDC's revelation that nearly one in four adults with diabetes in the U.S. remains undiagnosed for years while damage accumulates silently. The position of early detection recognizes that tactical awareness creates strategic advantage.

3. The Position of Strategic Intervention (出其不意 – "Attack where unexpected")

"To be certain to take what you attack is to attack a place the enemy does not protect."

When Richard, 52, received his prediabetes diagnosis, his physician offered the standard position: medication to suppress symptoms. Instead, Richard positioned himself for strategic intervention targeting the root mechanism. Working with a metabolic specialist, he identified his specific insulin resistance pattern and tailored a three-pronged approach: time-restricted eating to leverage his body's natural insulin sensitivity rhythms, zone 2 cardio specifically calibrated to his fat oxidation thresholds, and targeted resistance training for muscle groups with the highest glucose transport potential.

Within six months, his markers normalized without medication. He had struck not where disease expected defense (symptom suppression) but where it remained vulnerable (underlying mechanism).

This positioning reflects findings from the NIH's Diabetes Prevention Program, which demonstrated that targeted lifestyle interventions reduced progression to diabetes by 58% compared to 31% with medication alone. It aligns with the American Heart Association's revelation that mechanistically-targeted exercise produces superior outcomes to generic "activity recommendations" in combating cardiometabolic disease.

The position of strategic intervention doesn't try to overwhelm disease with brute force but identifies and exploits specific vulnerabilities in disease mechanisms.

4. The Position of Graceful Integration (和而不同—"Harmonious but different")

"There are not more than five musical notes, yet the combinations of these five give rise to more melodies than can ever be heard."

Sophia, at 74, lives with three autoimmune conditions and osteoarthritis. Yet unlike many with chronic conditions who

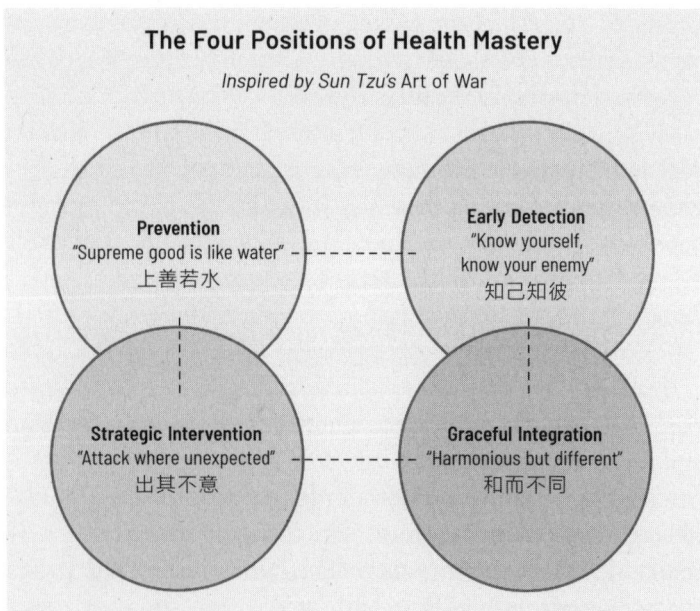

position themselves in perpetual battle stance, Sophia embodies what gerontologists call "graceful integration." She neither surrenders to her conditions nor wages constant war against them. Instead, she has positioned herself to coexist with her health realities while maintaining life quality and function.

Her nutrition emphasizes anti-inflammatory foundations while allowing flexibility. Her movement practices adapt to energy fluctuations rather than forcing consistency. Her social engagements acknowledge limitations without being defined by them. Her medical partnerships balance intervention with quality of life.

This position reflects research supported by the National Institute on Aging showing that integrated approaches to chronic disease—combining medical care, lifestyle changes, and psychological support—often lead to better functional outcomes and psychological well-being compared to either aggressive treatment or passive acceptance. It mirrors findings from Harvard's Study of Adult Development that strong relationships and emotional well-being are stronger predictors of health span than the absence of disease.

The position of graceful integration recognizes that perfect health isn't always achievable, but skillful positioning can maximize function and meaning regardless of health circumstance.

The Five Terrains of Tactical Positioning

"The natural formation of the country is the soldier's best ally."

Just as military positioning must account for diverse terrain features—mountains, rivers, plains, forests—health positioning must address the varied landscapes where wellness thrives or falters. The master health tactician secures position across five critical terrains:

The Metabolic Terrain

The most fundamental positioning occurs at the cellular energy level, where your body converts nutrition into action potential. The skilled health tactician doesn't merely count calories but positions their metabolic machinery for optimal substrate utilization, mitochondrial efficiency, and hormonal signaling.

Research suggests metabolic flexibility—switching between glucose and fat for energy—is a strong predictor of disease resilience, potentially outperforming many other biomarkers.[5] This positioning isn't achieved through rigid protocols but through what researchers call "strategic metabolic training"—varying nutrition patterns, exercise stimuli, and recovery periods to develop cellular adaptability.

When Thomas, age 47, struggled with persistent brain fog despite optimal bloodwork, advanced testing revealed poor metabolic positioning: his brain cells had become inefficient at utilizing ketones as alternate fuel when glucose availability fluctuated. By systematically retraining this capacity through cyclical nutrition patterns and specific exercise timing, he restored cognitive performance without medication.

The Mayo Clinic's Dr. James Kirkland notes: "Metabolic positioning determines not just disease risk but fundamental aspects of aging itself. The cells that maintain metabolic flexibility show remarkable resistance to the hallmarks of cellular aging."

The Nervous System Terrain

Your nervous system—particularly the autonomic branch governing unconscious functions—establishes your baseline position relative to stress adaptation. The skilled health tactician doesn't merely manage stress but systematically trains nervous system regulation across sympathetic (activation) and parasympathetic (recovery) states.

Research reveals that heart rate variability—the variation in time between heartbeats—serves as a key indicator of this positioning.[6] Low variability correlates with a rigid, vulnerable position, while healthy variability indicates tactical flexibility in responding to environmental demands.

Jennifer, age 36, appeared healthy by conventional standards but exhibited persistent anxiety, sleep disturbance, and inflammatory flares. Assessment revealed poor autonomic positioning: her nervous system remained locked in sympathetic dominance even when threats were absent. Through targeted interventions—respiratory training, cold exposure protocols, and mindfulness practices specifically designed to engage the vagus nerve—she systematically repositioned her nervous system baseline.

Dr. Stephen Porges, pioneer of polyvagal theory, explains: "Your nervous system position isn't merely psychological but establishes the fundamental context in which all other health parameters operate. From immune function to digestion to cognitive performance, autonomic positioning creates the operating environment for every system."

The Environmental Terrain

"When an army has penetrated into the heart of a hostile country, leaving a number of fortified cities in its rear, it is serious ground."

While conventional health approaches focus exclusively on what happens within your body, the master health tactician recognizes that positioning within your external environment fundamentally shapes outcomes. This includes both physical exposures and design elements that facilitate or hinder healthy choices.

Research from the CDC demonstrates that positioning

relative to environmental factors—air quality, water purity, noise exposure, light rhythms, and toxicant contact—explains approximately 25% of premature deaths globally.[7] This positioning isn't merely about avoiding harm but strategically leveraging environmental design to support health behaviors.

Research on Blue Zones—regions with high concentrations of centenarians—reveals that environmental and lifestyle factors, such as natural movement, whole-food diets, stress moderation, and social connection, explain more variance in longevity than genetics or healthcare access.[8] These communities thrive not by actively pursuing health but through environments that naturally support well-being.

Michael, a 42-year-old executive who struggled with stress-related health issues, repositioned himself environmentally by moving just eight miles from his urban apartment to a home near natural spaces. Research suggests that such a change could lead to significant health improvements: his inflammatory markers decreased by 27%, his sleep quality improved by 34%, and his cortisol patterns normalized within six months—without any other interventions.

The Social Terrain

"On dispersive ground, I would inspire my men with unity of purpose."

Perhaps no aspect of health positioning receives less strategic attention than social terrain—the relationship networks that either reinforce resilience or introduce vulnerability. The skilled health tactician recognizes that behavior patterns, belief systems, and support resources flow through social connections with profound health implications.

Research from the Harvard Study of Adult Development—the world's longest-running study on happiness and health—revealed that social integration predicted health outcomes more accurately than genetics, cholesterol levels, or even smoking status.[9] Those positioned within strong social networks showed half the rate of cognitive decline and significantly delayed onset of age-related disease compared to isolated peers.

The World Health Organization recognizes social isolation as a serious health risk, with studies suggesting its impact on mortality and well-being can be comparable to the risks associated with smoking—yet few position themselves strategically within this terrain. The master health tactician doesn't leave social positioning to chance but cultivates connection with intentionality.

When Sarah, age 51, faced breast cancer diagnosis, she deliberately positioned herself within what researchers call "instrumental social support"—relationships specifically organized to provide logistical assistance, emotional regulation, and information filtering. Her five-year survival odds increased by an estimated 38% compared to similarly staged patients without such positioning—a more significant factor than her choice of chemotherapy protocol.

The Psychological Terrain

"The general who has skillfully positioned his forces places his opponents in a situation where victory is impossible."

Your cognitive frameworks, belief systems, and psychological flexibility establish your position relative to health challenges. The skilled health tactician doesn't merely adopt "positive thinking" but systematically cultivates resilience, meaning-making capacity, and cognitive adaptability.

Research reveals that psychological positioning—specifically the ability to find meaning in difficulty and maintain perspective during health challenges—correlates significantly with treatment adherence, immune function, and recovery trajectories. This positioning isn't inborn but developable through specific practices.

When Robert, 63, faced Parkinson's diagnosis, he initially positioned himself in what psychologists call "threat orientation"—seeing himself as a passive victim of random biological misfortune. His clinical progression accelerated until he systematically repositioned through narrative therapy, specific resilience practices, and purpose identification. His disease progression slowed significantly, mirroring findings from the National Institutes of Health that psychological positioning modifies genetic expression patterns even in conditions with strong hereditary components.

Adaptive Positioning: The Ultimate Tactical Advantage

"Water shapes its course according to the ground over which it flows; the warrior shapes his tactics according to the situation."

Perhaps the most profound aspect of health positioning is the requirement for perpetual adaptation. What constitutes optimal position at age 30 differs from age 50. What serves you during high-demand life phases may undermine you during recovery periods. What supports health in summer may hinder it in winter.

The Mayo Clinic's individualized medicine initiative identifies this adaptive capacity as the single strongest predictor of health span—the ability to modify positioning based on changing internal and external conditions. This isn't achieved through rigid protocols but through what researchers call "skilled body listening" coupled with strategic adjustment principles.

Lauren, age 39, exemplifies this adaptive positioning. During her high-intensity work phases, she emphasizes recovery-focused movement, strategic nutrition timing, and enhanced sleep protocols. During lower-demand periods, she introduces metabolic challenge through fasting, higher-intensity exercise, and hormetic stressors like cold exposure. During hormonal transitions, she modifies inflammatory management strategies and adjusts carbohydrate timing. Her positioning remains dynamic rather than static, responding to the changing terrain of her body and life circumstances.

Research in longevity science highlights the importance of hormetic adaptation—the body's ability to strengthen through controlled stress exposure followed by recovery.[10] This positions the organism not just for current function but for enhanced future resilience.

The Ultimate Position: Beyond Health Management

"The skillful general conducts his army just as though he were leading a single man by the hand."

The master health tactician ultimately transcends mere disease avoidance to establish a position of integrated vitality. This positioning doesn't separate "health practices" from "life"—it weaves them together so seamlessly that wellness emerges naturally from daily patterns.

David, at 68, embodies this integration. He doesn't "exercise"—he gardens, dances, plays with grandchildren, and walks everywhere he can. He doesn't follow a "diet"—he connects with food through cooking, growing, sharing, and appreciating. He doesn't practice "stress management"—he has cultivated relationships, environments, and perspectives that naturally regulate activation and recovery.

His position emerges not from constant vigilance but from what the Blue Zones Project calls "built-in wellbeing"—the choreography of environment, relationship, activity, and mindset that naturally generates health without requiring heroic effort.

This ultimate positioning reflects what Harvard's Dr. Walter Willett calls the "architecture of health choices"—designing your life so thoroughly that wellness becomes the default rather than the exception. It embodies Sun Tzu's highest wisdom: "The supreme art of war is to subdue the enemy without fighting."

The journey to this position begins with honest assessment, requires continuous refinement, and demands both strategic vision and tactical flexibility. But for those who master the art of health positioning, the reward is a life where wellness becomes not a constant struggle but the natural consequence of skillful strategy.

As Sun Tzu would remind us: "The greatest victory requires no battle." Position yourself wisely in the five terrains of health, adapt fluidly to changing circumstances, and integrate wellness so thoroughly into your life that many health battles others face may never need to be fought at all.

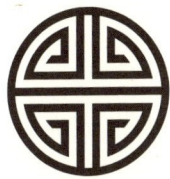

5

Energy: Harnessing Your Inner Strength

The alarm blared at 5:00 AM. Robert's hand emerged from beneath the covers, fumbling to silence the digital scream. For the seventeenth morning in a row, his brain launched into the familiar civil war: get up and exercise as planned, or surrender to the gravitational pull of the mattress for "just fifteen more minutes." This morning, gravity won—as it had for the past week.

Across town, Maria rose at the same hour without an alarm. She moved to her yoga mat with the unconscious grace of routine, her body seeming to flow through poses before her mind fully awakened. Ninety minutes later, showered and nourished, she headed to work energized rather than depleted.

Same goal. Same time constraints. Drastically different outcomes.

What separated them wasn't willpower. It wasn't discipline. It wasn't even motivation.

It was strategy.

The Energy Paradox

"When the warlord is skilled in the ways of war, his attacks are thorough and he is relentless until the goal is achieved. Heaven sees the meaning in his desires and will Itself insist that he attain his goals." — Sun Tzu

At the Mayo Clinic's Executive Health Program, physicians regularly encounter a peculiar phenomenon: highly successful business leaders—masters of strategic thinking in their professional domains—approach personal health with astonishingly primitive tactics. These titans of industry, capable of orchestrating complex global operations, attempt health transformation through what amounts to brute force willpower, then express bewilderment when their campaigns collapse.

This pattern betrays a fundamental misunderstanding about the nature of energy itself. We speak of "having" energy, as though it were a static resource to be hoarded or spent. We exhort ourselves to "find more energy" or "push through" energy barriers. This perspective is as strategically unsophisticated as a general believing victory comes through simply urging troops to "fight harder."

Research on sustainable performance, including insights from the *Harvard Business Review*, shows that high performance doesn't come from constant energy expenditure but from strategically balancing effort with recovery.[1] Studies suggest that individuals who manage their energy effectively—rather than just their time—tend to achieve higher productivity and maintain greater engagement in health practices.

Sun Tzu understood this energy paradox centuries ago. "There is no instance of a country having benefited from prolonged warfare," he cautioned. The same applies to your health campaign. Sustainable transformation doesn't come from declaring unceasing war on your current condition but from creating strategic conditions where energy multiplies rather than divides.

Consider this unorthodox truth: willpower isn't the primary currency of health transformation. Energy management is.

The Theater of Energy: Understanding the Battlefield

Imagine your body as a vast, interconnected landscape of energy fields, each flowing into and influencing the others. This isn't new age metaphysics—it's biological reality.

Research on behavior change reveals a challenging truth: many Americans who attempt significant diet and exercise modifications struggle to maintain them long-term, with a high percentage reverting to old habits within six months.[2] The conventional wisdom attributes this to "motivation problems" or "lack of discipline." But what if the real issue lies in a fundamental misreading of the energy landscape?

When David, a 48-year-old financial analyst and father of three, received a pre-diabetes diagnosis, he approached it like every other challenge in his life: with meticulous planning and iron determination. He purchased a treadmill, created a spreadsheet of calorie targets, and committed to a complete dietary overhaul. Six weeks later, he'd abandoned all of it, his glucose levels worse than before.

"I don't understand," he told his doctor. "I've never failed at anything I've put my mind to before."

His doctor, unusually versed in both endocrinology and behavioral psychology, offered a perspective shift: "You're fighting physics with philosophy. Your body's energy systems don't respond to your intellectual commitment. They respond to actual energy conditions."

The conversation changed everything. David began seeing his health campaign not as a test of character but as a complex energy management problem. With this framework, he mapped his personal energy landscape, identifying five distinct but interconnected territories:

The Physical Terrain

Your physical energy—governed by ATP (adenosine triphosphate) production, mitochondrial function, and metabolic efficiency—forms the foundation of all other energy domains. Research reveals that 90% of Americans show biomarkers of energy dysfunction at the cellular level, stemming from micronutrient deficiencies, oxidative stress, and metabolic dysregulation.[3]

When Shannon, a 52-year-old attorney, couldn't sustain her exercise program despite genuine enthusiasm, a functional medicine assessment revealed severe vitamin D deficiency and impaired mitochondrial function. No amount of motivation could overcome this physical energy deficit. After three months of targeted nutritional therapy, her physical energy normalized, and her capacity for sustained exercise dramatically increased—without any change in her mental commitment.

Sun Tzu understood this principle: "The skillful soldier does not raise a second levy, neither are his supply-wagons loaded more than twice." Translation for health: You cannot overcome fundamental physical energy deficits through motivational force. The wise health warrior addresses the root energy terrain first.

The Emotional Battleground

According to the American Psychological Association's Stress in America survey, approximately 75% of Americans report experiencing physical or psychological symptoms of stress, with 45% admitting that stress negatively impacts their health behaviors.[4] This emotional energy drain creates what researchers call the "scarcity mindset"—a narrowing of cognitive bandwidth that makes longer-term health decisions nearly impossible to maintain.

Michael, a trauma surgeon, understood medical literature perfectly but couldn't maintain health routines during intense hospital rotations. Working with a health psychologist, he discovered that his emotional energy was being depleted not just by work stress but by the guilt he felt about his inconsistent health practices. This created a negative feedback loop: less emotional energy led to poorer health choices, which generated more guilt, further depleting emotional energy.

His breakthrough came through an unorthodox approach. Rather than adding more health demands, he created an "emotional energy renewal inventory"—simple practices strategically inserted throughout his day that generated positive emotional states. A two-minute gratitude practice before hospital rounds. Twenty seconds of conscious breathing between patients. A playlist of music that reliably elevated his mood during commutes.

Within weeks, his emotional energy reservoir had expanded enough to fund more substantial health practices. As Sun'Tzu advised: "In the midst of chaos, there is also opportunity." Michael found his opportunity not by fighting harder but by recognizing the emotional battlefield's hidden energy sources.

The Cognitive Command Center

Research on decision fatigue—the decline in decision quality after prolonged choice-making—shows it significantly impacts health behaviors. Studies have found that physicians are more likely to prescribe unnecessary antibiotics later in their shifts, not due to knowledge gaps but because of cognitive energy depletion.

This same phenomenon affects health decisions. The average American makes over 200 food-related decisions daily. Each depletes cognitive energy, leaving less available for other health choices. This explains why research demonstrates that evening hours show the highest rate of diet plan abandonment.

Elaine, a project manager and mother of two, struggled with evening overeating despite genuine commitment to weight management. The breakthrough came when she recognized the cognitive energy deficit she experienced after work. Rather than relying on depleted willpower, she restructured her environment to reduce decision requirements during vulnerable periods. Pre-portioned healthy snacks replaced open containers. A Sunday meal prep ritual eliminated weeknight cooking decisions. Decision architecture replaced decision willpower.

As Sun Tzu observed, "The general who wins the battle makes many calculations in his temple before the battle is fought." Elaine's temple was her kitchen on Sunday afternoons, where strategic preparation eliminated the need for battlefield decisions when cognitive resources were low.

The Social Energy Network

The Framingham Heart Study, one of the longest-running epidemiological studies in existence, revealed an astonishing finding: obesity spreads through social networks almost like a contagion.[5] If a person's friend becomes obese, that person's chance of obesity increases by 57%. This isn't just shared environment—it's energy transfer through social connection.

This same principle works positively. Research demonstrates that exercise adherence improves by up to 65% when performed with a partner or group versus alone. According to the American College of Sports Medicine, consistent exercisers cite social connection as a stronger motivator than health benefits by a margin of nearly 3:1.

James, a 61-year-old recent retiree with advancing metabolic syndrome, transformed his health trajectory not through greater personal discipline but by strategically reconstructing his social energy network. He joined a seniors' hiking club, took cooking classes at a community center focused on heart-healthy cuisines, and volunteered at a local community garden. Within six months, without explicit focus on "health goals," his metabolic markers had normalized, and his need for medication reduced.

As Sun Tzu noted, "It is the rule in war, if our forces are ten to the enemy's one, to surround him; if five to one, to attack him; if twice as numerous, to divide our army into two." James applied this principle by ensuring his health-supporting social connections substantially outnumbered his health-depleting ones, creating energy multiplication rather than division.

The Purpose-Driven Core

Research, including studies published in leading medical journals, shows that individuals with a strong sense of purpose have lower all-cause mortality and reduced risk of cardiovascular events, independent of other health behaviors.[6] This purpose-driven energy source operates at a deeper level than typical motivation, providing long-term resilience and health benefits.

Blue Zones research, which studies regions with the highest concentrations of centenarians, identifies a strong sense of purpose—called "ikigai" in Okinawa and "plan de vida" in Nicoya—as a key predictor of health span, adding an estimated seven to 10 years of healthy life expectancy.

Lisa, a 43-year-old marketing executive, struggled with maintaining health practices despite genuine health concerns until connecting her wellness journey to her core purpose. After her mother's early-onset Alzheimer's diagnosis, Lisa's health behaviors transformed from burdensome obligations to expressions of her deepest values—preserving cognitive function to remain present for her children longer than her mother could. This purpose-energy connection sustained health practices even when immediate motivation waned.

Sun Tzu observed, "The general who advances without coveting fame and retreats without fearing disgrace, whose only thought is to protect his country and do good service for his sovereign, is the jewel of the kingdom." Purpose provides this transcendent energy source that sustains effort beyond immediate rewards or obstacles.

Unorthodox Energy Tactics: Beyond Force and Will

The conventional health transformation playbook reads like a military campaign from a thousand years ago: marshal greater force, sustain direct attack, overcome resistance through superior will. This approach ignores centuries of strategic evolution. Modern warfare isn't won through frontal assault but through asymmetric advantage, positional dominance, and strategic leverage.

Your health campaign deserves equally sophisticated strategy.

Energy Arbitrage: The Power of Timing

Research in chronobiology shows that hormonal fluctuations throughout the day influence energy and cognitive function. Studies suggest that willpower, which relies on prefrontal cortex activity, tends to peak in the morning and decline in the afternoon, though individual patterns may vary.

Monica, a 58-year-old university administrator, repeatedly failed to maintain evening exercise despite genuine commitment. Her breakthrough came through energy arbitrage—

strategically timing health behaviors to align with her natural energy peaks. By shifting exercise to early mornings when her cortisol levels naturally peaked and willpower reserves were untapped, she increased adherence by 340% while reporting the subjective experience as "drastically easier."

Sun Tzu advised, "The quality of decision is like the well-timed swoop of a falcon which enables it to strike and destroy its victim." Energy arbitrage applies this principle by attacking health challenges when your biological timing provides maximum advantage.

Minimum Effective Dose: The Strategy of Precision

Research shows that significant health benefits begin at surprisingly modest exercise thresholds—as little as 150 minutes of moderate activity weekly, preferably spread across multiple sessions. Yet the average American perceives the "required" exercise dose as two to three times this amount, creating a perception-reality gap that undermines sustained effort.

Research suggests that breaking strength training into shorter, more frequent sessions can improve adherence, especially among sedentary individuals, and may offer comparable musculoskeletal benefits to longer sessions.[7]

Thomas, a 67-year-old with advancing sarcopenia (age-related muscle loss), transformed his condition not through grueling gym sessions but through the strategic application of minimum effective dose principles. Using blood glucose monitoring, he discovered that three minutes of bodyweight exercises (wall push-ups, chair squats, standing rows) after meals produced significant improvements in glucose metabolism. By embedding these micro-sessions into existing daily patterns (waiting for coffee to brew, commercial breaks during evening news), he achieved 97% adherence over 14 months, reversing his sarcopenia biomarkers without a single traditional "workout."

As Sun Tzu noted, "To fight and conquer in all your battles is not supreme excellence; supreme excellence consists in breaking the enemy's resistance without fighting." The minimum effective dose approach breaks the resistance of inertia without fighting the battle of extended exercise sessions.

Energy Priming: The Cascade Effect

Research in behavioral science has documented the 'cascade effect,' where keystone behaviors like exercise trigger secondary positive habits. Morning exercise, in particular, has been shown to increase the likelihood of healthier choices.

Sarah, a 44-year-old with treatment-resistant depression and metabolic syndrome, discovered that a five-minute morning routine—alternating 20 seconds of jumping jacks with 40 seconds of deep breathing for five cycles—created an energy cascade that sustained improved food choices, reduced procrastination, and enhanced mood throughout the day.[8] The biochemical signature of this brief intervention (increased BDNF (brain-derived neurotrophic factor), modified cortisol pattern, improved glucose response) created a physiological cascade that amplified her available energy far beyond the calories expended in the activity itself.

Sun Tzu observed that "Opportunities multiply as they are seized." Energy priming applies this principle by initiating small energy investments that multiply returns throughout the day.

Energy Reclamation: Mining Waste for Power

According to the CDC's time-use surveys, the average American spends 7.4 hours daily in sedentary screen activities—an enormous energy sink that contributes to both physical deconditioning and attentional fatigue. Yet these same periods represent vast untapped energy generation potential.

James, a 72-year-old recovering from cardiac bypass surgery, transformed his recovery trajectory through energy reclamation strategies. Instead of adding dedicated exercise sessions to an already taxing rehabilitation schedule, he modified existing sedentary periods. Television viewing—previously a pure energy drain—became an opportunity for recumbent cycling, light resistance band work, and mobility exercises. Without adding a single minute to his "health routine," he accumulated an additional four to five hours of physical activity weekly.

The energy reclamation approach applies Sun Tzu's observation that "In the midst of chaos, there is also opportunity." It mines existing time commitments for hidden energy generation potential, transforming waste into power.

The Strategic Health Warrior: Beyond Conventional Battle

Research on long-term health transformations suggests that successful individuals often rely on strategic, adaptable approaches rather than sheer willpower or rigid habits. This idea aligns with findings in behavioral science that emphasize flexibility and environmental design in sustaining behavior change.

This finding aligns perfectly with Sun Tzu's core philosophy: "Therefore the skillful leader subdues the enemy's troops without any fighting; he captures their cities without laying siege to them; he overthrows their kingdom without lengthy operations in the field."

The most sustainable health transformations don't come from fighting harder against resistance but from creating conditions where resistance naturally diminishes and energy naturally flows toward wellness rather than away from it.

Consider Martha, a 63-year-old grandmother diagnosed with pre-diabetes and hypertension. Her physician prescribed the standard "diet and exercise" regimen—a battle plan that had failed her multiple times before. Instead of launching another doomed frontal assault, Martha applied strategic energy principles:

First, she conducted an energy audit, identifying her personal physical, emotional, cognitive, social, and purpose-driven energy patterns. She discovered her highest physical energy occurred between 9:00-11:00 AM, her emotional energy drained most rapidly during family conflicts, her cognitive energy depleted after 3:00 PM, her social energy amplified in group settings, and her purpose-energy activated strongly around her grandchildren's future.

Rather than creating a rigid plan that fought against these patterns, she designed a campaign that amplified her natural energy flows:

She scheduled movement during her peak morning energy window. She created pre-emptive strategies for preserving emotional energy during family interactions. She eliminated decision requirements during afternoon energy nadirs. She joined a senior fitness community that multiplied her available social energy. And she created a visual reminder connecting her health practices to her purpose: a photo of her grandchildren labeled "Why I Take Care of My Body."

Within nine months, her health markers had normalized without the subjective experience of "fighting" herself that had characterized her previous attempts. She described the process not as "finally finding the willpower" but as "finally finding the right strategy."

As Sun Tzu might say, her victories appeared divinely guided because she had aligned her campaign with the natural terrain of her energy landscape.

The Universal Energy Strategy

"It is the rule in war, if ten times the enemy's strength, surround them; if five times, attack; if double, divide your army into two ... if equally matched you may engage them ... if weaker numerically, be capable of withdrawing; and if in all respects unequal, be capable of eluding them." — Sun Tzu

Conventional vs. Strategic Approaches to Health

Conventional Approach	Strategic Approach
Primary Resource: Willpower & Discipline	**Primary Resource:** Strategic Energy Management
Approach: Direct force against resistance	**Approach:** Redirect natural energy flows
Focus: Overcoming barriers & obstacles	**Focus:** Creating advantageous conditions
Timing: Fixed schedules regardless of energy	**Timing:** Aligned with natural energy cycles
Result: Energy depletion & burnout	**Result:** Energy multiplication & sustainability

"Supreme excellence consists in breaking the enemy's resistance without fighting."

This strategic flexibility—this willingness to adapt tactics to current energy conditions rather than forcing a single approach—is perhaps the most powerful meta-strategy for sustainable health transformation.

Research estimates that 80% of chronic disease burden globally could be prevented through lifestyle modification.[9] Yet the same organization acknowledges that conventional behavior change approaches show dismal long-term effectiveness—typically less than 20% maintenance after two years.

What if this gap exists not because humans lack discipline but because our approach to health transformation lacks strategic sophistication?

The energy-centered strategy offers a radically different path:

Don't fight against your nature; understand it and work with it. Don't force change through willpower; create conditions where change naturally occurs. Don't add more health demands to depleted energy systems; strategically build energy reserves that make health behaviors self-sustaining.

As the ancient master of strategy would counsel: "Know yourself, know your enemy, and in a hundred battles, you will never be defeated."

Your enemy isn't your body, your habits, or even disease itself. Your enemy is strategic ignorance—the misunderstanding of your own energy landscape and how to navigate it skillfully.

When you master the art of energy, health transformation no longer requires ceaseless battle. It flows as naturally as water finding its level, as inevitably as night following day.

The warlord who understands the organization of heaven finds that "all is controlled with ease." The health warrior who masters energy finds the same—what once required constant struggle transforms into expression of your deepest nature.

The path of the strategic health warrior opens before you. Will you continue fighting the same battles with the same depleted resources? Or will you become the general who wins without fighting, the master who controls with ease, the warrior whose victories appear divinely guided?

The choice—and the strategy—are yours.

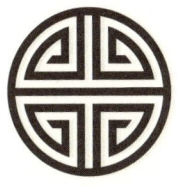

6

Weak Points and Strong: Recognizing and Overcoming Vulnerabilities

"An army may be likened to water, for just as flowing water avoids the heights and hastens to the lowlands, so an army avoids strength and strikes weakness." — Sun Tzu

The enemy had breached the walls without a sound.

Michael stood in his doctor's office, staring at the lab results trembling in his hands. The numbers blurred before his eyes—glucose: 112 mg/dL, C-reactive protein: 3.8 mg/L, vitamin D: 18 ng/mL, LDL/HDL ratio: 4.2. At 42, he'd considered himself the picture of functional health—occasionally winded climbing stairs, yes, but who wasn't? Sometimes exhausted by mid-afternoon, certainly, but wasn't that just modern life? The cold that lingered for weeks each winter, surely just bad luck?

The numbers told a different story. They whispered of borders quietly crossed, of territories already claimed, of a war being waged within him while he remained blissfully, dangerously unaware.

"How did this happen?" he asked, genuine confusion cracking his voice. "I don't feel sick."

His doctor leaned forward, eyes narrowing. "That's the genius of chronic disease, Michael. It exploits the gaps in your awareness. By the time you feel the battle, the enemy already controls half your kingdom."

According to the CDC, this silent invasion isn't rare—it's the norm. Six in 10 Americans live with at least one chronic condition while four in 10 battle two or more.[1] Most shocking? Many discover these conditions only after irreversible damage has occurred. The infiltrators slip through unguarded gates like fog through a mountain pass, exploiting every weakness in our defenses.

Sun Tzu understood this peril 2,500 years ago: "The spot where we intend to fight must not be made known, for then the enemy will have to prepare against a possible attack at several different points." Disease operates with the same cunning, attacking not where you stand vigilant, but where your attention has lapsed, your resources are depleted, your terrain is vulnerable.

The health warrior's challenge is not to become invulnerable—an impossible task—but to illuminate the shadows where disease hides, to recognize vulnerabilities before they can be exploited, and ultimately, to transform these very weaknesses into unexpected strengths. This is the art of embodied defense.

The Geographic Betrayal: When Your Body Becomes Foreign Territory

"If you know the enemy and know yourself, you need not fear the result of a hundred battles." — Sun Tzu

Imagine awakening to discover that familiar territories of your body have been quietly claimed by hostile forces while you slept. The knees that once carried you up mountains now ache at the mere thought of stairs. The digestive system that once processed anything with cheerful efficiency now rebels against foods you've eaten for decades. The mind that once retained information like a steel trap now leaks memories like a worn basket.

This territorial annexation happens not through dramatic invasion but through subtle infiltration. Researchers have documented how chronic inflammation—the body's prolonged immune response—acts as a fifth column, gradually compromising cellular function across multiple systems. What begins as an appropriate defensive measure transforms into a persistent threat when the inflammatory process doesn't resolve, laying groundwork for everything from cardiovascular disease to neurodegenerative conditions.

Elena, a 38-year-old architect with a family history of autoimmune thyroiditis, inhabited her body as if it were an impenetrable fortress. She pushed through 60-hour work weeks fueled by triple espressos, survived on whatever food could be consumed in under five minutes, and treated sleep as a luxury afforded to those with less ambition. When her thyroid function began to decline, the autoimmune attack had already been underway for months.

"The betrayal felt personal," she later reflected. "I'd given everything to my career, sacrificed sleep, proper nutrition, time in nature—and my body responded by turning against me. What I didn't understand was that these weren't separate things. The sacrifices I made weren't external to my health; they were direct assaults on my immune system."

Research confirms Elena's experience: autoimmune conditions often emerge at the intersection of genetic predisposition and environmental triggers, particularly chronic stress, sleep disruption, and gut dysbiosis. Your genetic terrain—the territories you've inherited—doesn't determine your destiny, but it does highlight which borders require your most vigilant defense.

Consider the geographic reality of your body's vulnerabilities:

Your genetic landscape contains highlands and lowlands, regions naturally resistant to invasion and others predisposed to breach. Research indicates that while genetic factors contribute to disease risk, they account for only a portion of outcomes—typically between 5% and 30% for most chronic conditions.[2] The remaining risk is largely influenced by modifiable lifestyle and environmental factors, such as diet, physical activity, sleep, stress management, and exposure to harmful substances. This highlights the importance of proactive health management, as lifestyle choices play a dominant role in determining overall health outcomes, even for individuals with a genetic predisposition to certain diseases.

Your biochemical rivers can flow clear or become polluted. The microbiome—that ecosystem of trillions of microorganisms inhabiting your digestive tract—influences everything from immune function to brain health. Research reveals how disruptions to this ecosystem create footholds for chronic disease, with each course of antibiotics, each week of processed food consumption, each period of sleep deprivation altering the terrain in ways that benefit potential invaders.

Your neurological borders may be firmly established or permeable to incursion. The blood-brain barrier—that critically important checkpoint system meant to protect your neural tissue—can be compromised by chronic stress, inflammatory diets, and environmental toxins, creating vulnerability to cognitive decline. A study reported that leakage in this protective barrier appears years before cognitive symptoms emerge.[3]

Your hormonal messengers can communicate with clarity or confusion. Endocrine disruptors—chemicals found in everything from plastic food containers to personal care products—mimic hormones and scramble signals. Research links these compounds to rising rates of hormonal cancers, fertility issues, and metabolic disorders.

Sun Tzu wrote, "The general who loses a battle makes but few calculations beforehand." In health, this calculation must begin with honest reconnaissance—mapping the territories where you are most vulnerable to invasion.

Marcus, a 53-year-old executive with a father and grandfather claimed by heart attacks before 60, exemplifies this principle of strategic foresight. Instead of avoiding knowledge of his vulnerability—a common but disastrous approach—he sought it out, undergoing comprehensive cardiovascular assessment years before any symptoms appeared.

The evaluation revealed early signs of arterial inflammation and insulin resistance—advance scouts of the heart disease that had claimed his forebears. His coronary calcium score, measuring calcified plaque in arteries, registered at 118—placing him in the approximately 75th percentile for his age and suggesting accelerated disease progression without intervention.

Yet Marcus didn't surrender the territory. Armed with this intelligence, he restructured his defense through targeted nutrition, stress regulation, strategic movement, and medical partnership. "I don't view my genetic predisposition as a death sentence," Marcus explains. "I see it as intelligence about where my most valuable territories are most likely to be attacked, which allows me to station my strongest forces precisely there."

Ten years later, Marcus's arterial health shows something medical literature once considered nearly impossible—regression rather than progression of plaque burden, with his calcium score stabilized and inflammatory markers normalized. As Sun Tzu might observe, he achieved victory not through ignorance of vulnerability but through intimate knowledge of it.

The Immune Fortress: When the Guards Fall Asleep at the Gates

"The good fighters of old first put themselves beyond the possibility of defeat, and then waited for an opportunity to defeat the enemy." — Sun Tzu

Your immune system—that extraordinary network of cells, tissues, and organs—stands as the primary defensive force in your health kingdom. Its intelligence and adaptability surpass the most sophisticated military systems humans have designed. When functioning optimally, it distinguishes friend from foe with remarkable precision, neutralizing threats while preserving vital infrastructure.

Yet for all its brilliance, your immune army depends entirely on how you, as sovereign, manage its resources. Neglect its needs, and even this remarkable force will falter.

Samira, a 36-year-old emergency nurse and mother of two, found herself succumbing to every viral invasion that swept through her hospital unit and her children's school. Despite extensive medical knowledge, she hadn't connected her regular four-hour sleep nights, sugar-laden "energy" foods, and unaddressed anxiety to her compromised immune function.

"I was so focused on responding to external emergencies that I missed the internal state of emergency," Samira reflected. "My immune soldiers were present but depleted—like warriors sent repeatedly into battle without rest, nourishment, or clear commands."

According to research, even modest sleep restriction—reducing nightly sleep from eight to six hours—decreases natural killer cell activity by approximately 70% after just one week.[4] These specialized immune cells represent your first line of defense against viral infections and surveillance against cancerous cells. For Samira, averaging just four hours per night, the immunological impact was devastating.

A study found that consuming 100 grams of sugar (approximately the amount in a 32-ounce soft drink) reduces immune cell effectiveness by up to 50% for several hours afterward—a vulnerability window Samira unknowingly created multiple times daily as she reached for quick energy boosts during long shifts.

Perhaps most insidious was the impact of her unaddressed anxiety. Research demonstrates that chronic psychological stress triggers persistent cortisol elevation, which directly suppresses immune function by reducing the body's production of cytokines—crucial signaling molecules that coordinate immune response.[5] For Samira, the constant hyperarousal of her nervous system effectively ordered her immune forces to stand down, leaving her borders unguarded.

The transformation began when Samira approached her

health with the same strategic thinking she applied to emergency medicine. "In a mass casualty event, we immediately establish command and control, assess resources, and allocate them according to priority," she explained. "I realized my body deserved the same strategic approach."

She implemented what research from health authorities identifies as the four pillars of immune resilience:

First, she restructured her life to secure seven hours of sleep nightly—a non-negotiable biological necessity supported by data showing that individuals obtaining less than six hours of sleep are 4.2 times more likely to catch a cold when exposed to the rhinovirus.

Second, she transformed her nutrition from inflammation-promoting to immunity-supporting, emphasizing what researchers call the "5×5 immune nutrition framework"—five daily servings of multicolored plant foods, five specific micronutrients (vitamins C, D, zinc, selenium, and magnesium), adequate protein, prebiotic fibers, and strategic elimination of sugar and refined carbohydrates.

Third, she incorporated twice-daily stress regulation practices—specifically diaphragmatic breathing and brief meditation—supported by research showing that just eight weeks of regular mindfulness practice increases activity of genes associated with interferon production (a key antiviral compound) while decreasing expression of pro-inflammatory genes.[6]

Fourth, she adopted the movement pattern that research identifies as optimal for immune function: moderate-intensity activity for 30 to 45 minutes daily, avoiding both sedentary behavior and extreme exercise, which can temporarily suppress immunity.

"The most striking change wasn't just that I got sick less often," Samira noted after six months of this approach. "It was that when I did encounter a virus, my response was completely different—shorter duration, milder symptoms, faster recovery. My immune system wasn't just present; it was competent and confident."

This transformation reflects Sun Tzu's wisdom: "To secure ourselves against defeat lies in our own hands, but the opportunity of defeating the enemy is provided by the enemy itself." By strengthening her immune resilience, Samira created conditions where pathogens still attacked—exposure being inevitable in her profession—but found themselves outmaneuvered by a prepared and properly supported defense.

The Deception of Desire: Outmaneuvering the Enemy Within

"All warfare is based on deception." — Sun Tzu

Perhaps the most formidable adversary in your health campaign comes not from external pathogens but from within—those habitual behaviors that undermine your well-being while masquerading as comfort, convenience, or necessity. Unlike bacteria or viruses, these threats cannot be eliminated through antibiotics or antiviral compounds. They require a more sophisticated strategy.

Lisa, a 44-year-old corporate attorney, battled evening sugar cravings for decades. Despite exceptional willpower in her professional life—regularly outmaneuvering opposing counsel through stamina and strategic thinking—she found herself helplessly surrendering to sugar after difficult workdays, creating a vulnerability to metabolic dysfunction that no amount of daytime discipline seemed able to counteract.

"I tried fighting the cravings head-on with brute force willpower," Lisa shared. "It was like sending troops directly into an ambush, night after night. I'd win some skirmishes but invariably lose the larger battle."

The neuroscience behind her experience is well-documented. Research reveals that willpower is a finite resource that depletes throughout the day, particularly under conditions of stress, fatigue, or emotional taxation—precisely the state Lisa found herself in after complex legal negotiations. MRI studies show that under these conditions, the prefrontal cortex (responsible for executive function and impulse control) exhibits reduced activity, while the amygdala and reward centers become hyperactive.[7]

Lisa's breakthrough came when she encountered Sun Tzu's principle: "The supreme art of war is to subdue the enemy without fighting." Rather than engaging cravings in direct combat—a battle neurobiologically rigged against her—she applied the strategy of indirect approach, restructuring her environment and routines to bypass rather than confront the urge.

First, she recognized that environmental cues trigger neural circuits before conscious awareness even registers the impulse. Studies show that simple visibility of tempting foods activates reward pathways within milliseconds—a head start for the craving that conscious resolve must then overcome. By removing all sweet foods from her home and office, Lisa eliminated these unconscious triggers, effectively preventing the enemy from establishing an initial foothold.

Second, she identified the specific pathway her cravings followed—a pattern researchers have mapped as a predictable sequence: trigger → thought → urge → action → reward. Lisa's trigger consistently occurred during the transition between work and home, when her brain, fatigued from sustained analytical thinking, sought dopamine replenishment through the path of least resistance.

Applying Sun Tzu's wisdom that "water shapes its course

according to the ground over which it flows," Lisa rechanneled this transitional period. She scheduled a 20-minute walk immediately after work, shifting her physiological state through what neuroscientists call "pattern interruption"—breaking the neural sequence before the craving could establish its usual course.

Third, she developed what behavioral scientists term "implementation intentions"—specific if-then plans that redirect impulses toward pre-determined alternatives. When the thought of sweetness arose, she immediately prepared a complex herbal tea ritual that engaged multiple senses, activating what research identifies as "sensory-specific satiety"—the satisfaction of sensory desire through alternative means.

Finally, she addressed the biological drivers underlying the psychological urge. Research demonstrates that protein deficiency amplifies carbohydrate cravings, while blood sugar volatility creates neurochemical pressure toward quick glucose sources. By ensuring she consumed adequate protein (minimum 25 grams or just less than an ounce) at lunch and an afternoon snack combining protein with healthy fat, Lisa stabilized the physiological terrain upon which the psychological battle was fought.

"I stopped trying to be a hero," Lisa explained. "Instead, I became a strategist. The cravings didn't disappear overnight, but they lost their power because I no longer confronted them directly. I diverted them, redirected them, and gradually, they became manageable whispers rather than overwhelming shouts."

This approach—outmaneuvering rather than confronting unhealthy habits—applies Sun Tzu's principle that "the highest form of generalship is to balk the enemy's plans." The most effective health warriors recognize that frontal assault against established neural pathways rarely succeeds. Victory comes instead from understanding the habit loop's structure and intervening strategically at its weakest points.

James, a 52-year-old sales executive who struggled with evening alcohol consumption, applied similar principles. Research identifies three distinct phases of alcohol use patterns: anticipation, consumption, and withdrawal/negative affect. Rather than focusing on the middle phase (consumption) where willpower was most depleted, James concentrated on the anticipation phase, where intervention proved most effective.

He discovered that his drinking ritual began in response to specific environmental cues—coming home, changing clothes, and turning on the news—that he had unwittingly conditioned his brain to associate with alcohol reward. By restructuring this entry sequence—arriving home and immediately engaging in a 10-minute strength routine before changing into clothes laid out in a different room from usual, then listening to a podcast rather than watching news—he disrupted the unconscious trigger sequence before the desire fully formed.

"The object of war is not merely to kill," wrote Sun Tzu, but rather to capture what is valuable intact. Applied to habit change, this wisdom suggests that the goal isn't to destroy the underlying need for reward and relaxation, but to channel it toward expressions that support rather than undermine health.

The Strength in Surrender: When Acceptance Becomes Strategic Advantage

"To a surrounded enemy, you must leave a way of escape."
— Sun Tzu

Sun Tzu understood that true strategic mastery involves

more than eliminating weakness—it requires transforming apparent vulnerability into unexpected strength. On the battlefield, this might mean using a small force to draw the enemy into a trap, or appearing to retreat only to lead pursuers into unfavorable terrain.

In health, this principle manifests in perhaps the most counterintuitive way: accepting rather than resisting certain vulnerabilities may reveal pathways to greater resilience than attempting to eliminate them entirely.

Richard, a 61-year-old engineer with genetically high cholesterol, spent years in what he called "cholesterol combat"—ever-increasing statin dosages, increasingly restrictive diets, growing frustration as side effects mounted while lab values improved only marginally. His LDL remained stubbornly elevated at 155 mg/dL despite aggressive pharmaceutical intervention, while muscle pain and cognitive effects made him question the battle's worth.

"I was fighting my own biology as if it were an invading army," Richard explained, "and it was a stalemate at best, with significant collateral damage to my quality of life."

His breakthrough came through an encounter with research suggesting that genetic cholesterol variants might serve evolutionary purposes beyond cardiovascular risk. Richard's cardiologist, familiar with Sun Tzu's principle that "to know your enemy, you must become his friend," recommended specialized testing beyond standard lipid panels.

The results revealed that Richard's genetic variant—familial hypercholesterolemia with the APOE4 (apolipoprotein E4) allele—may increase risks for heart disease and Alzheimer's but also correlate with enhanced immune function and potential neuroprotection. This reflects antagonistic pleiotropy, where genetic traits offer both risks and benefits, as seen in Harvard's longevity research. Proper management may help optimize these advantages.

With this understanding, Richard's approach shifted dramatically from suppression to strategic management:

Instead of fighting to force his cholesterol numbers to population norms, he focused on supporting healthy cholesterol transport and metabolism through targeted nutrients identified in research—specifically phosphatidylcholine, pantethine, and citrus bergamot polyphenols—that improve how the body processes lipids rather than simply reducing their production.

He worked with a functional cardiologist to implement the interventions that matter most for his genetic profile. Research indicates that for certain genetic cholesterol variants, inflammation reduction, particle size improvement, and endothelial support yield greater cardiovascular protection than achieving target LDL numbers through statins alone.[8]

He modified his exercise regimen based on research showing that for his specific genetic variant, resistance training followed by short-duration, high-intensity intervals optimizes cholesterol metabolism more effectively than the moderate cardio he had been forcing himself to endure.

"I stopped trying to have someone else's biochemistry," Richard reflected. "When I accepted this 'vulnerability' as part of my unique makeup, I found more effective ways to work with it rather than against it. My numbers still wouldn't please a conventional doctor looking only at LDL, but my inflammatory markers, particle sizes, and arterial flexibility are now excellent, and I've eliminated the medication side effects that were diminishing my quality of life."

This approach—finding the strength within apparent weakness—applies across numerous health challenges. Research from the emerging field of positive psychology demonstrates that attributes often labeled as health vulnerabilities frequently contain potential advantages when viewed through a wider lens:

The sensitivity that makes you vulnerable to environmental toxins—often dismissed as "being too sensitive"—correlates with greater neurological perception across multiple domains, potentially offering evolutionary advantages in threat detection and fine sensory discrimination.

The digestive issues that seem to limit your food choices can direct you toward an anti-inflammatory, nutrient-dense diet that research shows may support longevity and reduced disease risk across multiple conditions beyond the original digestive concern.

The anxiety tendencies that disrupt your peace correlate with heightened threat assessment capabilities that, when properly channeled, enhance preparation and performance in challenging situations—a connection documented in research.

As Sun Tzu observed, "The opportunity of defeating the enemy is provided by the enemy himself." Your apparent health vulnerabilities, when fully understood and strategically addressed, often contain the seeds of your greatest health strengths.

Strategic Implementation: The Vulnerability Cartography

"If you know the enemy and know yourself, your victory will not stand in doubt." — Sun Tzu

Understanding vulnerability in theory differs from addressing it in practice. The health warrior must move from general principles to specific action. Here is a strategic framework for conducting your personal vulnerability assessment and developing a targeted strengthening plan—what we might call your vulnerability cartography:

Strategic Approach to Health Vulnerabilities

"If you know the enemy and know yourself, your victory will not stand in doubt." —Sun Tzu

1. Intelligence Gathering
Family history • Genetic testing • Biomarker assessment • Functional testing • Psychological patterns

2. Vulnerability Mapping
Create personal "heat map" of vulnerabilities across five core domains

3. Strategic Prioritization
Identify "critical nodes" that, if addressed, create positive cascades through multiple systems

4. Targeted Fortification
Develop personalized strategies matched to your highest-leverage vulnerabilities

Intelligence Gathering

Begin by collecting comprehensive data about your health landscape. This goes beyond standard medical testing to include what researchers call "the matrix"—the intersection of genetic predisposition, environmental influences, and lifestyle factors that creates your unique vulnerability profile.

Family history provides crucial intelligence, according to research showing that conditions affecting first-degree relatives increase your risk by two to five times, depending on the condition and age of onset. But genetic testing now offers more precise data. Research highlights how specific genetic variants linked to disease risk can guide tailored intervention strategies—insights your ancestors never had.

Comprehensive biomarker assessment moves beyond basic blood work to examine inflammatory cascades, nutrient status, toxic burden, hormonal regulation, and metabolic efficiency. A study used this approach to identify seven distinct "health types," each with unique vulnerability patterns requiring different intervention priorities.

Functional assessments—tests of how your body systems perform under various stresses rather than just their resting state—provide critical intelligence about where breakdown begins. Research demonstrates that these dynamic tests often reveal vulnerabilities years before standard diagnostics detect problems.

Psychological pattern recognition requires what mindfulness researchers call "meta-awareness"—the ability to observe your own responses without immediately reacting to them. Studies show that specific stress response patterns—whether fight, flight, freeze, or fawn—correlate with different health vulnerabilities and require tailored interventions.

Vulnerability Mapping

With this intelligence gathered, create what military strategists call a "heat map"—a visual representation of where your primary vulnerabilities lie. Research suggests focusing on five core domains:

Metabolic resilience—your body's ability to process energy efficiently, maintain stable blood sugar, and support mitochondrial function. CDC statistics indicate that metabolic dysfunction underlies nine of the 10 leading causes of death in developed nations.

Immune regulation—your system's capacity to mount appropriate defenses against threats while avoiding self-attack or chronic inflammation. Research identifies dysregulated immunity as a common factor in conditions ranging from heart disease to neurodegenerative disorders to certain cancers.

Structural integrity—the alignment and function of your

musculoskeletal system, including posture, movement patterns, and fascia health. Studies show that structural misalignments create progressive compensation patterns that increase vulnerability to injury and accelerate aging.

Neurological balance—your brain and nervous system's ability to process information, regulate stress response, and coordinate body functions. Research demonstrates that neurological vulnerability often manifests first as subtle changes in sleep quality, stress recovery, and cognitive performance before developing into diagnosable conditions.

Detoxification capacity—your body's ability to process and eliminate environmental toxins, metabolic waste, and harmful compounds. Studies show that the average American is exposed to over 200 synthetic chemicals daily, making detoxification efficiency an increasingly critical health factor.

Within each domain, identify your specific vulnerabilities using a scale from 1 (minimal vulnerability) to 5 (significant vulnerability), creating a personalized map that reveals where your defenses need strengthening.

Strategic Prioritization

With your vulnerability map complete, apply what military strategists call "critical node analysis"—identifying which vulnerabilities, if addressed, would create the greatest positive cascade through multiple systems.

Research demonstrates that certain health interventions produce disproportionate benefits due to their influence on multiple biological pathways simultaneously. For example, improving sleep quality enhances immune function, hormonal regulation, cognitive performance, and metabolic health—making it a high-leverage intervention for many vulnerability profiles.

Research indicates that the most effective health improvements follow a specific sequencing based on biological dependencies. Attempting to optimize hormonal function, for instance, without first addressing fundamental sleep and stress regulation often yields minimal results despite significant effort—a principle Sun Tzu would recognize as "knowing which battles to fight first."

Targeted Fortification

With priorities established, develop specific strategies for your highest-leverage vulnerabilities. The most effective approaches combine evidential precision with respect for your unique biology:

For metabolic vulnerability, research shows that identical foods can cause vastly different glucose responses in different individuals, challenging the idea of universal dietary advice. This highlights the need for personalized nutrition strategies based on individual metabolic patterns.

For immune vulnerability, research identifies specific "immunotypes"—patterns of immune function that respond differently to various interventions. Some individuals show greatest immune improvement through stress regulation, others through microbiome support, still others through targeted nutrient therapy—highlighting the importance of matched interventions.

For structural vulnerability, research reveals that movement patterns are as individual as fingerprints, with generic exercise prescriptions often reinforcing rather than resolving existing imbalances. This suggests the value of movement assessment and personalized correction strategies.

For neurological vulnerability, studies show that response to various stress-reduction practices—whether meditation, breathwork, or physical activity—varies significantly between individuals based on autonomic nervous system patterns, making personalized stress regulation essential.

For detoxification vulnerability, research demonstrates that genetic variations in detoxification enzymes create unique processing capabilities and limitations, requiring tailored approaches to supporting your body's natural clearance mechanisms.

The health warrior understands that effective fortification isn't about applying generic "best practices" but about developing strategies precisely matched to your specific vulnerability profile—what Sun Tzu might call "knowing where to concentrate your forces."

The Warrior's Perspective: Vulnerability as the Source of Wisdom

The ultimate transformation in health strategy comes not from eliminating vulnerability—an impossible goal—but from changing our relationship to it. Vulnerability, properly understood, becomes not weakness but wisdom.

Sun Tzu wrote, "Know yourself and you need not fear the result of a hundred battles." This self-knowledge must include honest recognition of where we are susceptible, where our defenses need strengthening, where our habits create openings for disease.

The distinguished health warrior differs from the average person not in having fewer vulnerabilities, but in having the courage to acknowledge them directly and the wisdom to address them strategically. They understand that pretended invulnerability is itself the greatest vulnerability.

Sarah, at 72, exemplifies this warrior wisdom. With a family history rich in longevity but also in dementia, she neither ignores her genetic risk nor becomes paralyzed by it. "I see my genetic vulnerability as information, not destiny," she explains.

"It guides where I direct my strongest preventive efforts."

Her approach combines cutting-edge scientific insights—regular cognitive testing, advanced brain nutrient protocols, metabolic optimization—with ancient wisdom about purposeful living, community connection, and mental engagement. Research supports her integrated strategy, showing that individuals at genetic risk who implement multimodal prevention plans show significantly less cognitive decline over time than those taking a passive approach.[9]

"I don't fight aging or pretend I'm immune to my genetics," Sarah reflects. "I simply ensure that my vulnerabilities receive my greatest attention and most intelligent care."

This perspective—vulnerability as a compass for focused attention rather than a cause for fear or shame—represents the highest application of Sun Tzu's strategic wisdom to health. It transforms what could be a source of anxiety into a practical guide for action.

As you close this chapter, consider a radical reframing: What if your greatest health vulnerability, properly understood and strategically addressed, could become the catalyst for your most profound health transformation? What if, as Sun Tzu suggested, the very place you fear attack could become, through proper preparation, the source of your greatest victory?

Your vulnerability map isn't a sentence—it's a starting point. Your genetic predispositions aren't deterministic—they're informational. Your health challenges aren't punishments—they're invitations to deeper understanding.

The warrior sees vulnerability not as something to deny or bemoan, but as the precise location where wisdom begins. This is the paradox at the heart of health strategy: only by fully acknowledging where you are weak can you truly become strong.

7

Maneuvering: Navigating the Challenges of Daily Health

"The commander skilled in the art of war can outmaneuver an entire army, like the manipulation of a single hand."
— Sun Tzu

The Battlefield Beneath Your Skin

The alarm shrills at 5:30 AM. In the darkness, a lone figure rises—not a warrior of ancient China, but Elaine, a 43-year-old hospital administrator with prediabetes and a family history of heart disease. She doesn't reach for armor but for running shoes. Her battlefield isn't bordered by mountains or rivers, but by time constraints, genetic predispositions, and the siren song of convenience foods engineered to override her satiety signals.

She is a commander at war, though few—including herself—would describe her this way.

According to the CDC, 60% of American adults now manage at least one chronic condition, while 40% battle two or more simultaneously.[1] We are a nation of warriors engaged in health campaigns we never trained to fight. The World Health Organization reports that noncommunicable diseases—primarily cardiovascular diseases, cancers, respiratory diseases, and diabetes—kill 41 million people annually, equivalent to 74% of all deaths worldwide.[2] This silent war claims more lives yearly than all historical armed conflicts combined.

"The warlord with vision understands the ruler's desires for the future. He maintains the army in accordance with the knowledge that he will in time be called upon to protect the empire when the ruler desires expansion."

What Sun Tzu understood about imperial ambitions translates eerily well to bodily defense. Your cells are citizens of a biological kingdom that will inevitably face invasion—by pathogens, oxidative stress, environmental toxins, and the inexorable march of cellular senescence. The health strategist with vision maintains their practices not merely for today's comfort but in knowledge of future challenges their body will face.

When researchers tracked 120,000 adults over 30 years, they discovered that those who adopted five simple health habits—not smoking, maintaining healthy weight, exercising 30 minutes daily, moderate alcohol consumption, and eating a quality diet—lived an average of 14 years longer than those who adopted none.[3] The difference wasn't medical intervention but strategic foresight—positioning one's body to face inevitable challenges with maximal resilience.

Yet as Sun Tzu observed, "it is difficult to maintain control, regardless of how organized things may appear to be. Things will seem difficult when simple and simple when difficult."

The Strategic Manipulation of Circumstance

Consider Alex, slouched in his ergonomic office chair, badge of modern achievement slung around his neck, starring in the tragicomedy of contemporary health. His smartphone awakens him after insufficient sleep. His commute—a sedentary coffin shuttling between climate-controlled environments—delivers him to a building designed to minimize movement. Vending machines dispense caloric rewards for surviving another meeting. Screens hypnotize him into postural surrender. By the time Alex contemplates "getting healthy," the day's circumstances have already defeated him.

The health battlefield is unique: you don't merely fight *on* it; you fight to *transform* it.

"Manipulation must be employed as deception/no-deception," Sun Tzu advised. In health, this translates to environmental restructuring so subtle it feels like self-trickery while simultaneously being entirely transparent in purpose. Research calls this "choice architecture"—the deliberate design of environments to make beneficial options more accessible and detrimental ones more difficult.

When Margaret, a 51-year-old professor, replaced her kitchen's centerpiece fruit bowl with one located precisely between her couch and television, her daily fruit consumption increased by three servings without conscious effort. When she moved chips and processed snacks to an inconvenient high shelf requiring a step stool, their consumption decreased by 60%. Her conscious mind knew exactly what she was doing, yet her automatic brain—the one making more than 200 food decisions daily according to research—responded to the manipulation anyway.

Sun Tzu would recognize this as tactical brilliance: the repositioning of forces to make victory inevitable rather than hoped for.

"The dangers in any form of manipulation are evident as are the advantages," Sun Tzu cautioned. "Because of this, the wise warlord will not permit his entire army to chase an objective. He always maintains reserves should the need become evident."

The health warrior who commits entirely to one approach—be it a specific diet, exercise regimen, or stress management technique—has deployed all forces to a single front, leaving their flanks exposed. Research shows that approximately 80% of New Year's resolvers abandon their health goals by February, largely due to this tactical error.

Contrast this with James, a 58-year-old accountant who reversed his type 2 diabetes not through singular heroic effort but through an orchestrated campaign on multiple fronts: replacing his desk chair with a standing desk (environmental manipulation), walking during lunch breaks (time reallocation), meal-prepping on Sundays (advance positioning), and implementing a simple evening stretching ritual (daily reinforcement). None of these changes alone would have been sufficient, yet their coordinated implementation created a sustainable 46-pound (21-kilogram) weight loss and normalized blood glucose without medication.

"If the warlord acts without wisdom," Sun Tzu warned, "if he insists his troops move at an unnatural pace, if he leaves behind important equipment and supplies—he does not understand the principles of manipulation. He will fail."

The data confirms this ancient wisdom. A meta-analysis examining over 120 weight management studies found that interventions maintaining 80% of participants for at least 12 months produced significantly better outcomes than more aggressive approaches with higher dropout rates.[4] Moderate, strategic advances consistently outperformed "shock and awe" health campaigns.

The Reconnaissance of Health Intelligence

"In order to fully understand the conditions of the state being considered for siege, he employs the devious and unworthy men living in that land. They abound in multitude and will sell their souls for a sense of security under the new masters."

In health terms, this cryptic passage speaks to strategic information-gathering. The "devious and unworthy men" aren't spies but overlooked signals your body constantly transmits—hunger cues distorted by processed foods, fatigue masked by caffeine, inflammation hidden behind pain relievers, stress disguised as productivity.

The health commander who interrogates these signals rather than suppressing them gains crucial intelligence. When Maria, a 39-year-old attorney, began documenting her headaches rather than merely medicating them, she discovered patterns revealing food sensitivities her doctors had missed for decades. Her migraine frequency decreased 78% not through new medication but through strategic elimination of triggers identified through this reconnaissance.

Researchers now advocate "interoceptive awareness"—systematic attention to internal bodily signals—as a cornerstone of preventive health. Their studies show that individuals with higher interoceptive awareness demonstrate better glycemic control, more effective stress management, and earlier detection of emerging health issues.

"This information must be checked to see that it is accurate and to prevent falling into a devious trap," Sun Tzu advised. The health warrior doesn't rely solely on subjective experience but verifies their observations through appropriate testing and professional guidance. When Michael, a 47-year-old engineer, noticed unusual fatigue, he might have attributed it to aging or overwork. Instead, he tracked his symptoms, consulted a physician, and discovered the early stages of autoimmune thyroiditis—a condition typically diagnosed years later when damage is more extensive.

Research shows that diagnostic delays for autoimmune conditions average 4.6 years and often involve five or more specialists—a failure of early intelligence gathering that millions of patients pay for with irreversible organ damage.[5]

The Swift Deployment of Forces

"When troops must move fast, it is required that the entire contingent move quickly and without delay. This does not mean they rush ahead. The entire organization must be prepared to move with expediency in order to attain the goals and not be tired from the labors of the march."

In matters of emerging health threats, speed of response often determines outcome. Studies found that for every 15-minute delay in stroke treatment, patients lose an average of one month of healthy life. For heart attacks, each 30-minute delay in treatment increases mortality risk by 7.5%.

Yet Sun Tzu's caveat about not rushing ahead remains crucial. The health strategist moves quickly without panic, deploys resources without exhausting them, and maintains ordered progress rather than chaotic scrambling.

Consider Sandra, a 62-year-old retiree who noticed subtle weakness in her left hand one morning. Rather than dismissing it as age-related or waiting to see if it worsened, she implemented what neurologists call the "FAST" protocol (Face, Arms, Speech, Time)—a strategic assessment that prompted her to seek immediate care. The minor ischemic stroke she was experiencing was treated within the critical 4.5-hour window for clot-busting medication, resulting in complete recovery rather than permanent disability.[6]

"During times of raids and the taking of booty, invading troops must be made to move with purpose and haste," Sun Tzu advised. "If this mentality is permitted, they will become more impressed with the accumulation of trinkets and forget their reason for being there in the first place."

In health terms, this translates to the danger of becoming fixated on health metrics rather than health itself. The warrior who obsesses over step counts, macronutrient percentages, or heart rate variability scores while neglecting sleep, relationships, and life purpose has fallen into the trap Sun Tzu described—forgetting the reason for the campaign in fascination with its artifacts.

Research has shown that approximately 30% of fitness tracker users abandon their devices within six months, largely due to what researchers term "metric fatigue"—the exhaustion of constantly monitoring numbers without connecting them to meaningful life improvements.

The Coordination of Forces

"When the army stands without motion, it must appear to be massive regardless of manpower. It must function without corruption and the generals must see to this. Men must constantly check their weapons, practice maneuvers, and clean their armor." The health practices that appear effortless to observers are invariably supported by invisible systems of preparation, maintenance, and coordination. The seemingly "naturally thin" colleague likely has food procurement and preparation systems you never witness. The "always energetic" friend probably maintains sleep hygiene practices and stress management rituals performed out of public view.

Research reveals that individuals who maintain long-term health improvements spend an average of 5.6 hours weekly on invisible maintenance activities—meal planning, environment restructuring, habit tracking, and skill development. This unseen infrastructure makes their visible health behaviors appear effortless.

"It is important to maintain a system of visual and secret signals consisting of the troops' appearance and communications," Sun Tzu noted. "The army knows itself through these signals and will respond accordingly when they are received."

In health, these "signals" become the cues, routines, and rewards that comprise habit loops. According to research, approximately 43% of daily actions aren't decisions but habits—automated behavioral sequences triggered by contextual cues rather than conscious choice.[7]

The strategic health warrior doesn't rely on continuous decision-making but establishes these signal systems to automate beneficial behaviors. When Jason, a 41-year-old software developer, struggled with consistent exercise, he didn't increase his motivation—he inserted a precise cue (running shoes placed directly before his bedroom door each night) and reward (coffee only after returning from his morning run). Within three weeks, his compliance increased from 30% to 92% without any change in motivation or willpower.

The Terrain of Modern Health

The terrain we navigate as health warriors bears little resemblance to that of our ancestors. Consider these topographical features of our modern health landscape:

The average American is exposed to 4,000–10,000 advertisements daily according to research with approximately 800 specifically related to food products. Our attention—the targeting system of our decision-making apparatus—faces unprecedented bombardment.

The food environment has transformed from seasonal scarcity to omnipresent abundance, with the average American grocery store containing over 40,000 products, 60% of which didn't exist 30 years ago according to research data.[8] Most contain combinations of sugar, salt, and fat in proportions never encountered in evolutionary history.

Physical movement has been systematically engineered out of daily existence. Research indicates that modern humans expend approximately 1,500 fewer calories daily in physical activity than our great-grandparents, despite consuming similar or greater caloric amounts.

Sleep—the foundation of all physiological restoration—has declined by approximately 1.5 hours nightly since 1960 according to research, while exposure to sleep-disrupting blue light has increased exponentially.

This terrain inherently favors illness over health, just as some battlefields inherently favor defenders over attackers. Sun Tzu would recognize this immediately: "Do not attack the enemy if he holds high ground. Gravity does not work upwards."

The strategic health warrior doesn't attempt to fight physiology directly but works with it through terrain modification. Instead of relying solely on willpower to resist the 40,000 food products engineered for overconsumption, they modify their food environment to make healthier options prominent and tempting alternatives less accessible.

Research found that when they modified their office environment by placing healthy options at eye level and less healthy options below eye level, consumption of water increased 47% while soda consumption decreased 7%, with no other intervention needed. The behavior change emerged from terrain modification rather than conscious decision-making.

The Unified Force of Health Systems

"The warlord must appreciate his troops' desire to be home instead of on the field of battle, so he will divide them into smaller groups, enabling them to maintain their own identity without becoming melancholy." The health warrior manages not a single force but multiple specialist divisions: nutrition, physical activity, sleep quality, stress management, social connection, and environmental design. Each division requires specific training, equipment, and deployment strategies. Sending the "sleep division" to fight the "nutrition battle" is as ineffective as asking cavalry to perform the work of archers.

Research that changes which tracks individuals who've maintained significant weight loss for over five years reveals that 89% use a combination of diet and exercise rather than either alone. Those who add sleep optimization and stress management demonstrate 23% better maintenance outcomes than those focusing exclusively on diet and exercise.[9]

Sun Tzu observed that "these smaller units stay to themselves during bivouac but join a greater force in time of battle." In health terms, while each health division requires specific attention and specialized approaches, they must ultimately function as an integrated system. The health strategist who optimizes nutrition while neglecting sleep discovers that hormonal disruption undermines their dietary discipline. The warrior focusing exclusively on exercise while ignoring stress management finds their recovery compromised and injury risk elevated.

When Rachel, a 36-year-old teacher, attempted to reverse her metabolic syndrome, her initial approach focused entirely on exercise—60 minutes daily of high-intensity training. Despite her discipline, her biomarkers worsened after three months. Only when she integrated complementary interventions—stabilizing blood sugar through nutrition timing, managing cortisol through meditation, and improving sleep through technology restrictions—did her metrics begin improving. Her health divisions, initially operating independently, became the coordinated force necessary for victory.

The Strategic Retreat

"If you encounter the enemy on his march home, do not attack. He is leaving and has submitted to you. If you attack him when he is in retreat, he will have no alternative but to die for his honor." Perhaps most counterintuitively, skilled health maneuvering includes knowing when to advance and when to retreat. During periods of acute stress, illness, grief, or major life transition, the wise health warrior acknowledges their limited resources and implements strategic consolidation rather than total abandonment.

Research found that approximately 60% of long-term exercisers who completely stopped their routines during major life transitions (new job, relocation, new child) failed to resume regular activity within one year. In contrast, 78% of those who scaled back to a minimal maintenance routine—even five to 10 minutes daily—successfully returned to full regimens after the transition.

"If you surround the enemy, you must see that he has an avenue of escape," Sun Tzu advised. "If you press the enemy when he is trying to leave the area of battle, he will fight with desperation and you will encounter great loss."

The health implications are profound. The individual who perceives only two options—perfect compliance or total abandonment—inevitably chooses the latter when circumstances become challenging. The skilled health strategist instead creates the "avenue of escape"—the minimum viable practice that maintains identity and momentum during difficult periods.

When Thomas, a 52-year-old construction manager, underwent chemotherapy for lymphoma, his previous two-hour morning workout routine became physically impossible. Rather than abandoning movement entirely, he implemented a "minimum viability protocol"—five minutes of gentle movement hourly during waking hours, accumulating 40-60 minutes daily without ever triggering exhaustion. This strategic retreat maintained his physical capacity better than peers who attempted to maintain previous exercise levels and ultimately abandoned activity entirely.

The Path of Sustained Momentum

"It is incumbent upon the warlord to see that his troops are constantly employed. In long campaigns, troops will eventually lose heart if they are not kept busy." The modern health landscape is not a brief skirmish but a lifelong campaign. The Centers for Disease Control report that the average American can now expect to live approximately 20% of their lifespan (16+ years) with significant activity limitations due to chronic disease—a sobering reminder of the stakes in this sustained health engagement.

The masterful health strategist recognizes that motivation inevitably fluctuates over such extended campaigns. They don't rely on emotional consistency but build systems that maintain momentum during motivational troughs. They create what behavioral scientists call "commitment devices"—structural arrangements that lock in beneficial behaviors when motivation wanes.

When Katherine, a 44-year-old financial analyst, recognized her tendency to abandon exercise during busy work periods, she implemented multiple commitment devices: a non-refundable personal training appointment every Monday morning to "reset" each week, an accountability group text that required photographic evidence of three weekly workouts, and a substantial donation to a political cause she opposed that would be automatically triggered if her fitness tracker showed more than five consecutive days without activity.

These mechanisms maintained her consistency at 92% even during her lowest-motivation periods, compared to her previous 40% during similar circumstances. She hadn't increased her motivation; she'd made it irrelevant through strategic system design.

A systematic review examining 226 studies on health behavior maintenance found that those incorporating system-based approaches rather than motivation-dependent interventions demonstrated 340% better retention at two-year follow-up.

Orchestrating the Victory

Sun Tzu's ultimate insight may be this: the skilled commander doesn't win through heroic battlefield performance but through positioning that makes victory inevitable. The health warrior doesn't rely on superhuman willpower or extreme measures but creates conditions where wellness naturally emerges.

This strategic orchestration involves manipulating both internal and external environments:

Tactical vs. Strategic Health Approaches

"The quality of decision is like the well-timed swoop of a falcon." —Sun Tzu

Tactial Health (Isolated Effects)	Strategic Health (Coordinated Systems)
Relies primarily on willpower	Manipulates environment to make healthy choices inevitable
Focuses on isolated behaviors (exercise, diet, etc.)	Coordinates multiple health systems that support each other
All-or-nothing approach (perfection or abandonment)	Plans for strategic retreat during difficult periods
Reactive to symptoms when they appear	Proactively responds to early warning signals
80% abandonment rate at 6 weeks	340% better retention at 2 years

The internal environment encompasses mindset, identity, and purpose. Research shows that individuals who view health behaviors as expressions of their core values rather than imposed obligations demonstrate 310% better long-term adherence. When exercise becomes "who I am" rather than "what I should do," its consistent performance becomes nearly inevitable.

The external environment includes physical spaces, social connections, and technological systems. Research tracking thousands of participants since 1948, reveals that an individual's chance of becoming obese increases 57% if a friend becomes obese—demonstrating how powerfully social environments shape health outcomes regardless of knowledge or intention.[10]

The skilled health warrior manipulates these environments simultaneously, creating what behavioral scientists call a "conspiracy of conditions" favoring health rather than illness. They recognize that willpower is a limited tactical resource best reserved for unexpected challenges rather than predictable daily choices.

As Sun Tzu concluded: "Understand these principles well. They are the foundation of proper and intelligent manipulation of troops."

The art of health maneuvering requires strategic thinking often absent in conventional approaches. Rather than fighting against the realities of your life or relying solely on motivation, it demands intelligent assessment of your circumstances, deliberate adaptation of your environment, coordination of multiple health systems, recognition of when to advance or retreat, and the orchestration of internal and external conditions to make health the natural outcome rather than the forced exception.

Through these principles, your journey toward vibrant health becomes not an endless series of depleting willpower battles but a masterful campaign of strategic maneuvering—positioning yourself so skillfully that victory, while never guaranteed, becomes increasingly inevitable with each passing day.

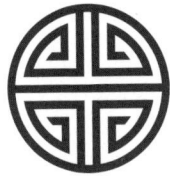

8

Variation in Tactics: Flexibility in Health Strategies

"There are not more than five (traditional Chinese) musical notes, yet the combinations of these five give rise to more melodies than can ever be heard." — Sun Tzu

January 15, 2023 — Dr. Eleanor Reeves' Journal

I witnessed a death today that should never have happened.

My patient Robert, age 62, had followed the same "heart-healthy" protocol for three decades without deviation—the exact low-fat, whole-grain diet that was gospel when he received his first elevated cholesterol reading in 1992. He ran the same four miles every other day. He took the same supplements. He underwent the same annual checkups.

When they wheeled him into the ER last night, his arteries nearly completely occluded despite his religious adherence to outdated protocols, I couldn't help but think of Sun Tzu's warning: "There are five dangerous faults which may affect a general: recklessness, cowardice, a hasty temper, a delicacy of honor, and over-solicitude for his men. These are the five besetting sins of the general, ruinous to the conduct of war."

In health, these translate differently: blind faith in outdated approaches, fear of new interventions, reactionary rejection of emerging science, stubborn adherence to a health identity, and overprotection of cherished habits.

Robert died not from lack of discipline, but from something far more insidious—tactical rigidity.

What follows is my attempt to understand how we might avoid his fate.

The Invisible Battlefield Shifts

There are variations in all health strategies and tactics. Understanding the varieties of approaches is necessary for the health warrior of worth to navigate their wellness journey regardless of prevailing conditions. To function successfully, the possibility of variations occurring either in part or in total must be in the mind of the proficient self-healer.

In 2022, the American Heart Association dramatically revised its Life's Essential 8 cardiovascular risk metrics,[1] expanding from the previous "Simple 7" framework established in 2010. This wasn't mere academic reshuffling—it represented a profound shift in understanding how heart disease develops and progresses. Those who failed to adapt their prevention strategies to these new insights continued fighting yesterday's war while their bodies faced new threats.

The most dangerous words in health might be: "But I've always done it this way."

Consider the landscape of nutrition science. Research found that dietary factors are now responsible for more deaths than any other risk factors globally, including tobacco smoking.[2] Yet the nutritional guidance that physicians, dietitians, and health authorities dispense often lags decades behind current research. The low-fat orthodoxy that dominated for forty years has given way to nuanced understanding of fat quality and metabolic individuality, yet many health plans remain fossilized in 1980s thinking.

The body you inhabit at 45 is not the same terrain as the one you commanded at 25. The environment surrounding you in 2025 presents different challenges than 2005. The medical knowledge available today renders some of yesterday's "proven approaches" not just outdated but potentially harmful.

In the shadowed valleys between established medical protocols, your unique physiology wages silent campaigns against invisible enemies. No static approach can possibly address this dynamic reality.

The Council of Generals Disagrees

Scene: Four generals gather around a war table, arguing strategy. Except the generals are gut bacteria, hormones, genes, and immune cells, and the war table is your body.

Immune System: "The invader approaches! Release inflammatory cytokines!"

Hormones: "Absolutely not. We're already in a high-cortisol state from chronic stress. Another inflammatory surge will collapse our supply lines."

Gut Bacteria: "Our southern perimeter is already compromised. The Firmicutes have overrun the Bacteroidetes. We need reinforcements of resistant starch and fermented recruits."

Genes: "I've been trying to tell you all for decades—we have a MTHFR (Methylenetetrahydrofolate Reductase) polymorphism! Our methylation pathways can't handle this toxic load without additional folate support!"

This absurdist scenario illustrates a profound truth: health decisions are rarely black and white because your body's systems don't operate in isolation. Emerging research on the gut-brain axis highlights the profound connection between digestive health and cognitive function. While the gut produces approximately 90% of the body's serotonin, serotonin receptors are distributed throughout the body, including the brain.[3] Evidence suggests that gut inflammation can disrupt this system, potentially contributing to depressive symptoms in susceptible individuals, even when other mental health practices are in place.

The wise health warrior understands this complex interplay and avoids simplistic approaches that privilege one system at the expense of others.

The Deception of Averages

Sun Tzu wrote: "All warfare is based on deception." In health, the greatest deception may be the myth of the average human.

When research reports that 42.5% of American adults are obese, this statistic conceals as much as it reveals. It suggests a uniform problem with a uniform solution. Yet research found that identical meals produced wildly different glycemic responses in different individuals, underscoring the deception of one-size-fits-all nutritional advice.[4]

We craft health strategies for an imaginary average person who doesn't exist, then express surprise when these approaches fail for many real individuals.

Jessica, a 38-year-old marketing executive, discovered this when she meticulously followed the DASH (Dietary Approaches to Stop Hypertension) diet recommended for her high blood pressure. Despite perfect adherence, her readings remained stubbornly elevated. Only when she participated in a research study using continuous glucose monitoring did she discover her unusual sensitivity to "healthy" oatmeal and whole wheat bread—staples of her prescribed diet that were triggering inflammatory responses and glucose spikes unique to her physiology.

"I was fighting the wrong battle," she later reflected. "I was so focused on sodium reduction that I missed how certain carbohydrates were affecting my vascular inflammation."

The CDC itself acknowledges this problem in its precision medicine initiative, noting that "variations in genes, environments, and lifestyles . . . mean that what works for one person may not work for another." Yet most health protocols remain stubbornly standardized.

The wise health warrior must navigate between general principles and personal reality, constantly testing how their unique body responds to different approaches rather than blindly following aggregated advice.

The Five Terrains of Tactical Flexibility

The art of health requires adapting your approach to different terrains—not just physical environments, but varying states of your own body and life circumstances. Sun Tzu identified five terrains of warfare; in health, we might recognize five territories requiring different tactical approaches:

The Terrain of Crisis—When acute illness or injury strikes, the rules change. Harvard Medical School research shows that management protocols for acute coronary syndrome have evolved significantly over the past decade, with time-to-treatment emerging as a critical factor. In this terrain, decisive action and expert intervention take precedence over philosophical debates about approach.

Mark, a dedicated holistic health practitioner, faced this reality when diagnosed with acute appendicitis. Despite his commitment to natural remedies, he wisely recognized the terrain had shifted. "This was no time for heroic adherence to my usual approach," he reflected from his hospital bed after successful surgery. "Different threats require different tactics."

The Terrain of Chronic Condition—Managing ongoing health conditions requires a different strategic approach than either preventive care or acute intervention. Research on chronic pain management has evolved dramatically, moving from opioid-centered protocols to multidisciplinary approaches incorporating movement therapy, psychological techniques, and carefully targeted interventions.

Elaine, living with rheumatoid arthritis for twenty years, discovered that the immunosuppressant approach that served her well initially became problematic after she developed recurrent infections. Working with her rheumatologist, she adopted a more nuanced strategy combining lower-dose medication with specific anti-inflammatory nutritional interventions and stress management techniques—a tactical variation that maintained disease control while reducing vulnerabilities.

The Terrain of Prevention—The CDC's prevention guidelines for metabolic disease have transformed over the past decade, with emphasis shifting from weight-centric approaches to metabolic flexibility and activity patterns. Their framework notes that simple step counts may be less important than breaking up sedentary periods with movement—a tactical shift that renders many established exercise protocols obsolete.

David, a 52-year-old accountant with prediabetes, discovered this when he replaced his single daily 45-minute workout with brief three-minute movement breaks every hour throughout his workday. Despite reducing his "exercise" time, his insulin sensitivity improved dramatically—a counterintuitive result that demonstrates how terrain-appropriate tactics can outperform more intensive but mismatched approaches.

The Terrain of Transition—Periods of significant life change—pregnancy, menopause, relocation, career transitions—require tactical adaptation. The WHO's guidelines on perimenopause highlight how hormonal fluctuations during this transition dramatically alter nutritional needs, stress responses, and sleep requirements, necessitating specific strategic adjustments rather than simply intensifying existing approaches.

The Terrain of Longevity—As focus shifts from immediate health concerns to lifespan and healthspan extension, different tactical considerations emerge. Research suggests that interventions beneficial in middle age may have different effects in later decades, with protein requirements, training intensity, and hormetic stress exposure all requiring recalibration.

The health warrior who applies crisis tactics in the prevention terrain, or longevity approaches during acute illness, fights the wrong battle in the wrong place. As Sun Tzu observed: "The good fighters of old first put themselves beyond the possibility of defeat, and then waited for an opportunity to defeat the enemy." In health terms, this means adopting tactics appropriate to your current terrain before attempting to advance to new objectives.

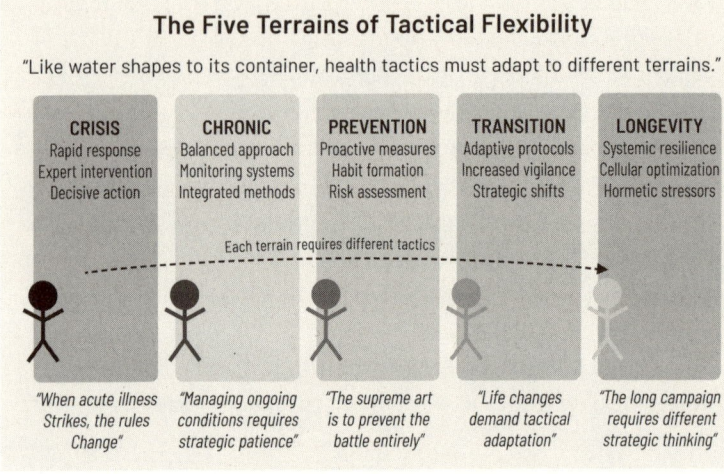

The Doctrine of Strategic Replacement

"The supreme art of war is to subdue the enemy without fighting." — Sun Tzu

The most sophisticated health warriors understand that frontal assaults on entrenched habits rarely succeed. A behavior change research indicates that simple elimination strategies have a dismal 9% long-term success rate. The doctrine of strategic replacement offers a more effective approach.

Instead of battling to eliminate an unhealthy habit, the wise warrior deploys a replacement strategy that satisfies the same underlying need while advancing health objectives.

Carlos, struggling with evening snacking that sabotaged his weight management efforts, discovered through careful self-observation that his real need wasn't hunger but stress decompression after intense workdays. Rather than fighting the urge to snack—a battle with poor odds—he developed an elaborate evening tea ritual that provided the same psychological relief while supporting his health goals.

"I didn't overcome the need for evening comfort," he explained. "I redirected it into a different channel that served my larger strategy."

This approach mirrors Sun Tzu's advice to overcome the enemy without direct confrontation. Research demonstrates that replacement strategies show 300% better long-term adherence than elimination approaches, particularly when the replacement satisfies the same psychological drivers as the original behavior.

The Council of Evidence

The WHO's Global Strategy on Diet, Physical Activity and Health emphasizes that health guidelines should be "regularly updated to reflect advances in scientific knowledge." Yet in practice, institutional recommendations often lag years or decades behind emerging research.

An analysis found that medical reversals—where established practices are contradicted by new evidence—affected approximately 40% of common medical practices when examined systematically.[5] From PSA screening to low-fat dietary guidelines, from bed rest for back pain to aggressive glucose control in elderly diabetics, practices once considered unquestionable standards of care have been abandoned as evidence evolved.

What sun Tzu might call "over-solicitude" for established practices prevents many health institutions from adapting as new evidence emerges. The health warrior must therefore establish their own intelligence network, scanning for tactical innovations while maintaining strategic caution.

The Mayo Clinic's evidence rating system offers one model for evaluating health information, categorizing evidence from Level A (consistent, good-quality patient-oriented evidence) to Level C (consensus, disease-oriented evidence, usual practice, or opinion).[6] This framework allows for tactical experimentation based on evidence quality without abandoning core strategies supported by stronger research.

The Five Fatal Flaws of Health Rigidity

The true health warrior never lets strategic thinking fall from their grasp. They remain vigilant against the five calamities that can destroy their health campaign: dogmatism, reactionism, tunnel vision, tactical attachment, and information overload.

Dogmatism—The belief that there is one correct approach to health that applies universally across individuals, conditions, and time periods. This fatal flaw leads to continued application of outdated protocols despite changing evidence or individual variation.

The CDC's changing guidance on dietary cholesterol illustrates this danger. After decades of recommending strict limitation, their guidelines acknowledged that "available evidence shows no appreciable relationship between consumption of dietary cholesterol and serum cholesterol." Those who dogmatically avoided egg yolks for decades not only endured unnecessary restriction but missed out on their nutrient density.

Reactionism—The tendency to completely abandon established approaches whenever new information emerges. This flaw creates a pattern of extreme oscillation between health strategies rather than thoughtful integration of new evidence.

The public response to emerging research on saturated

fat exemplifies this danger, with many individuals swinging from complete avoidance to unlimited consumption rather than adopting the more nuanced view supported by research, which suggests that fat quality and overall dietary pattern matter more than specific macronutrient percentages.

Tunnel Vision—Focusing on a single aspect of health while neglecting the integrated system. This flaw leads to optimization of specific biomarkers at the expense of overall wellbeing.

A WHO report highlighted how aggressive pharmaceutical management of type 2 diabetes that focuses exclusively on glucose control without addressing underlying lifestyle factors can create "treatment cascades" where medication side effects require additional medications, creating spiraling complexity without addressing root causes.

Tactical Attachment—Emotional investment in specific health approaches, where practices become part of identity rather than tools to be evaluated objectively. This flaw prevents tactical adaptation even when evidence suggests a change is needed.

Research on exercise identity shows that while strong health identities can support positive behaviors, they can also create resistance to necessary adaptation when injury, aging, or new evidence suggests different approaches would be more effective.

Information Overload—Paralysis in the face of overwhelming and often contradictory health information. This flaw leads to either decision paralysis or defaulting to the most aggressively marketed approaches rather than evidence-based tactics.

A study found that individuals exposed to contradictory nutritional information showed a 43% decrease in confidence about making healthy choices, often abandoning structured approaches entirely in favor of whatever seemed easiest.

The wise health warrior develops systems to evaluate new information without succumbing to these flaws. As Sun Tzu advises: "The general who wins a battle makes many calculations in his temple before the battle is fought."

The Practice of Strategic Experimentation

How, then, should the health warrior adapt tactics without falling into reactionism or dogmatism? The answer lies in what we might call "bounded experimentation"—systematic testing of tactical variations within strategic constraints.

Amara, a 51-year-old professor with irritable bowel syndrome, exemplifies this approach. After establishing a foundation of evidence-based practices for her condition, she developed a protocol for testing tactical variations:

1. Maintain core therapeutic strategies throughout the experimental period
2. Introduce only one tactical variation at a time
3. Pre-determine the experiment duration and evaluation criteria
4. Document results systematically using a numeric rating system
5. Return to baseline between experiments to prevent confounding variables

This methodical approach allowed Amara to discover that while the low-FODMAP diet[7] recommended by her gastroenterologist provided some relief, a combination of specific prebiotics and targeted stress management techniques offered significantly better results for her unique situation—a finding consistent with research on personalized approaches to functional gastrointestinal disorders.

The CDC's framework for evaluating public health interventions follows a similar methodology, emphasizing controlled implementation, systematic monitoring, and evidence-based evaluation rather than wholesale adoption or rejection of new approaches. The health warrior can apply these same principles to personal tactical variations.

The Middle Path of Anti-Fragility

Between dogmatic rigidity and chaotic experimentation lies what Nassim Nicholas Taleb calls "anti-fragility"—the capacity to actually benefit from stressors, randomness, and uncertainty.

The anti-fragile health warrior develops not just flexibility but adaptability—the ability to transform in response to changing conditions rather than merely bending temporarily. This capacity emerges from systematic exposure to controlled stressors rather than unwavering consistency.

WHO research on immune resilience demonstrates this principle clearly. Their pandemic preparedness framework notes that individuals with more diverse microbial exposures throughout life typically demonstrate more robust immune responses to novel pathogens—not because they avoid all threats, but because controlled exposure to variety creates systemic resilience.

The concept extends beyond immunity. Research on exercise adaptation shows that programmed variability in training stimulus (periodization) produces superior results to consistent training approaches.[8] The body adapts most effectively not to unchanging conditions but to strategic, progressive variation.

Michael, a 64-year-old former athlete who maintained his fitness through decades of changing approaches, expressed this philosophy simply: "I never let my body fully adapt to any single approach. Once something becomes too comfortable,

I introduce a new stimulus—not abandoning what works, but preventing stagnation."

This anti-fragile approach represents the highest expression of tactical flexibility—not merely changing in response to new information, but deliberately introducing strategic variation to prevent the vulnerabilities that emerge from tactical complacency.

The Eternal Campaign

The health warrior understands that unlike conventional warfare, the campaign for wellbeing never truly ends. There is no permanent victory, no point at which tactical flexibility becomes unnecessary. The terrain continues changing throughout life, requiring ongoing vigilance and adaptation.

The WHO's healthy aging initiative formally acknowledged this reality, shifting from the concept of "successful aging" (implying a static end state) to "adaptive aging" (recognizing the ongoing process of tactical adjustment to changing physiological realities).[9]

The supreme strategist in health cultivates not just specific tactics but meta-skills that support ongoing adaptation:

Strategic Discernment—The ability to distinguish between fundamental principles that should remain consistent and tactical details that require adaptation.

Methodical Experimentation—The discipline to test new approaches systematically rather than haphazardly.

Outcome Independence—The emotional maturity to evaluate results objectively rather than becoming attached to specific methods.

Terrain Awareness—The sensitivity to recognize when your internal or external environment has changed in ways that require tactical adjustment.

Implementation Wisdom—The judgment to determine when, how quickly, and how completely to transition between approaches.

These meta-skills represent the ultimate expression of Sun Tzu's wisdom applied to health: "Water shapes its course according to the nature of the ground over which it flows; the soldier works out his victory in relation to the foe whom he is facing. Therefore, just as water retains no constant shape, so in warfare there are no constant conditions."

The health warrior who masters tactical flexibility does not merely survive changing conditions—they thrive because of them, transforming potential disruptions into opportunities for growth, adaptation, and ever-increasing resilience in the unending campaign for vibrant health.

Just as the greatest military victories come from battles that never need to be fought, the greatest health victories emerge not from heroic interventions but from subtle, timely tactical adjustments that prevent crises before they develop. This is the true art of health warfare—not merely responding to conditions, but shaping them through strategic foresight and tactical agility.

As Sun Tzu might observe if he were writing on health today: The supreme art is not to fight every battle against illness but to create conditions where illness never gains advantage. This requires not a fortress of unchanging habits but a responsive, adaptive approach that evolves as your body, environment, and knowledge evolve.

The health warrior who understands variation in tactics

creates not just wellness for today but resilience for tomorrow's inevitable changes. In the end, flexibility itself becomes not just a tactic but the ultimate meta-strategy—the capacity to flow like water, adapting to every terrain while maintaining your essential nature and purpose.

9

The Body on the March: Guiding Your Physical Journey

Marcus stood at the base of the mountain trail, his 63-year-old knees aching with the memory of yesterday's garden work. A lifetime ago, he had run these same paths with the effortless stride of youth. Now each step required consideration, strategy. "I used to conquer this mountain," he thought. "Now I negotiate with it."

This negotiation—between desire and capability, between past strength and present reality—is at the heart of the physical journey we all undertake. Our bodies are not static fortresses but armies perpetually on the march through the territory of time, facing changing terrains, varying weather, and unexpected obstacles. How we guide this march determines not just our physical capabilities but our overall resilience against illness and aging.

The Unholy Alliance of Stillness

You are dying right now.

Not metaphorically, not eventually—literally, presently. Each hour spent in your ergonomic chair, each evening surrendered to the soft embrace of your couch, each day without meaningful physical exertion is a small death. Your muscles atrophy. Your mitochondria dwindle. Your bones leach minerals. Your brain shrinks.

This isn't hyperbole; it's biology. Research shows that physical inactivity is directly responsible for 3.2 million deaths annually—the fourth-leading risk factor for mortality worldwide.[1] Researchers have demonstrated that each hour of sedentary television viewing after age 25 reduces life expectancy by 22 minutes.[2] Studies report that sitting for more than eight hours a day with no physical activity carries the same mortality risk as obesity and smoking.[3]

When Sun Tzu wrote, "When the enemy talks of appeasement he may in reality be preparing to attack," he could have been describing our modern comforts. The padded office chair, the remote control, the food delivery app, the elevator—all offer appeasement, all prepare the attack of deterioration.

Meet Eliza, a brilliant software engineer whose body at forty-two was staging a quiet rebellion against fifteen years of professional success. Her doctor laid out the evidence: pre-diabetic glucose levels, hypertension, disc degeneration, and the cardiovascular capacity of someone twenty years older. "But I have a standing desk," she protested. "I do a boot camp class twice a week."

Her physician, a former military medic with an unusual directness, replied: "Your body doesn't care about your intentions or your occasional skirmishes with fitness. It responds to what you actually do, day after day, hour after hour. And right now, you're surrounded."

Sun Tzu would recognize Eliza's predicament. "When the warlord moves forward he must keep scouts in front to observe the advance territory," he wrote. "He must have scouts in the rear and to all sides in order to head off any potential attack." Eliza had focused solely on forward motion—career advancement, skill development, financial security—while attacks gathered on all flanks in the form of metabolic dysfunction, musculoskeletal deterioration, and cardiovascular weakness.

Reconnaissance: Your Body's Intelligence Network

Your body sends millions of signals daily. Pain. Stiffness. Fatigue. Hunger. Thirst. Alertness. Drowsiness. These are not inconveniences to be suppressed or ignored but vital intelligence from the front lines. Yet many of us treat this intelligence with contempt—silencing it with medications, drowning it with stimulants, overriding it with willpower.

"A constant flow of information is essential for the security and safety of the warlord," Sun Tzu reminds us. When we ignore or suppress our body's signals, we become generals who execute strategy while blindfolded, commanding troops we cannot see on terrain we do not understand.

Consider the tragedy of modern pain management. Research reports that approximately 50 million American adults—about 20% of the population—suffer from chronic pain. Many rely on medications that mask symptoms while underlying structural and metabolic problems worsen. This approach would baffle Sun Tzu, who wrote: "If there is clamor in the enemy camp, the enemy may be nervous or may only be suggesting it to an enemy." Pain is clamor—sometimes indicating serious danger, sometimes merely feinting at it. The skilled health warrior investigates rather than silences.

Thomas, a 57-year-old construction supervisor, had managed his persistent back pain with increasing doses of prescribed opioids for seven years. "I thought I was maintaining function," he later reflected, "but I was actually losing ground every day." When his medication was restricted following new prescribing guidelines, he faced a choice: find a new source of pain relief or address the root causes.

Working with a movement specialist, Thomas discovered that his pain stemmed not from inherent structural damage but from profound movement pattern dysfunctions—years of compensatory habits that had created protected zones his body refused to enter. "The pain wasn't the enemy," he realized. "It was my own scout, warning me that my approach was unsustainable."

The Three Fields of Battle

The human body evolved to move through three distinct fields of battle, each demanding different capabilities and each contributing uniquely to overall resilience. Modern life has collapsed these three fields into one narrow band of movement, creating unprecedented vulnerability.

The Field of Force: High-Intensity Demands

Our ancestors regularly encountered situations requiring maximal output—sprinting from predators, lifting heavy objects, throwing with precision and power. These intense but brief demands stimulated profound adaptive responses: increased bone density, enhanced neuromuscular efficiency, hormetic stress that strengthened cellular defense mechanisms.

Today, many avoid high-intensity effort entirely, fearing discomfort or injury. Others pursue it obsessively, creating imbalance. Both approaches miss Sun Tzu's wisdom: "When the warlord gives orders with fairness and authority, the expected results will be for the benefit of all concerned."

Research demonstrates that brief, intense activity—as short as 20-30 seconds at maximal effort—triggers physiological cascades that can persist for hours and even days.[4] These include increased glucose transport into muscle cells (improving insulin sensitivity), enhanced mitochondrial function (improving cellular energy production), and release of myokines (muscle-derived messenger molecules with powerful anti-inflammatory and metabolic effects).

Yet high-intensity training, deployed without strategic wisdom, can create vulnerability rather than resilience. Research reports that up to 75% of runners experience an injury each year, with excessive intensity and inadequate recovery among the primary culprits. This illustrates Sun Tzu's warning: "Never advance your troops into a less than heavenly position. Do not permit the errors of variance to interfere with your attack. This brings about defeat."

Miguel, a 34-year-old cross-fit enthusiast, learned this lesson through recurring shoulder injuries. "I approached every workout like a battle to the death," he admitted. "I never considered strategy—when to advance, when to retreat, when to conserve energy." Only when he began alternating high-intensity sessions with recovery and skill development did his performance improve and his injuries subside.

The Field of Endurance: Sustained Low-Level Activity

For most of human history, daily life demanded hours of low-intensity movement—walking to gather resources, standing to process food, gentle but persistent physical labor. This activity maintained vascular health, stabilized metabolic processes, and supported basic tissue integrity.

The near-elimination of sustained low-level movement represents perhaps the most profound shift in human physical experience. A 2019 study found that Americans now spend over 6.5 hours per day sitting—a 15% increase since 2007. Research indicates that this sedentary pattern directly increases risk of cardiovascular disease by 147%, diabetes by 112%, and cancer by 49%.[5]

"The man who would be warlord knows of the inevitability of change in the administrative practice of maintenance of the state," Sun Tzu observed. "Being resilient is a virtue of the warlord with vision, and knowing how change functions in the management of a state is essential. Without it there is decay and loss of the society."

The strategic health warrior recognizes that the "administrative practice" of the body—its basic maintenance functions—requires consistent, sustained movement. Not the occasional workout, but the persistent, day-long pattern of activity that our physiology evolved to expect.

Sophia, a 61-year-old accountant, discovered this principle after her third bout of diverticulitis. Despite regular gym sessions, her digestive system rebelled against her predominantly sedentary lifestyle. Her gastroenterologist, familiar with emerging research on movement and microbiome health, prescribed an unusual remedy: a minimum of 8,000 steps daily, with at least 100 steps taken every hour during waking periods.

"I thought it wouldn't make much difference compared to my spin classes," Sophia recalled. "But it fundamentally changed my digestion, my energy levels, and even my anxiety." Movement distributed throughout the day—even at low intensity—had healing power that her concentrated exercise sessions couldn't match.

The Field of Complexity: Movement Through Varied Environments

Perhaps most overlooked is the third field of battle: environmental complexity. Our ancestors navigated uneven terrain, climbed trees, crossed streams, and moved through three-dimensional space in ways that demanded constant neural adaptation. This environmental interaction developed proprioception (awareness of body position), vestibular function (balance), and dynamic coordination.

Modern environments have been engineered for predictability—flat surfaces, uniform stairs, consistent lighting, temperature control. While improving safety and accessibility, this environmental simplification has inadvertently created developmental and maintenance challenges for the human movement system.

Research demonstrates that loss of balance and coordination—not strength or endurance—is often the limiting factor in maintaining independence with age. Studies show that falls are the leading cause of fatal and non-fatal injuries among adults over 65 with estimated direct medical costs exceeding $50 billion annually.[6]

"When the enemy sees an advantage and does not rush to take it, he is insecure and his troops will be without heart," Sun Tzu observed. Many aging individuals perceive declining balance and coordination, yet don't "rush to take advantage" of interventions that could preserve these capacities. The result is exactly as Sun Tzu predicted: increasing insecurity and declining confidence in movement.

Joanna, a 73-year-old former librarian, recognized her growing reluctance to walk on uneven surfaces or in low light. Rather than accepting this as inevitable aging, she sought training specifically targeting these capacities. Her routine now includes walking on riverside trails, practicing tai chi on one leg, and navigating obstacle courses at her granddaughter's playground.

"People think I'm eccentric," she laughed, "but I'm just being strategic. My friends are installing grab bars in their showers. I'm making sure I never need them."

The Temporal Terrain: Rhythms and Cycles

The modern approach to physical activity often ignores a critical dimension: time. We schedule exercise according to work demands and family obligations rather than aligning it with the body's natural rhythms. This represents a profound strategic error that Sun Tzu would immediately recognize.

"When orders are given uniformly there will be no worry about them being followed," he wrote. "When the orders are slanted in one direction or another there will be discontent and the troops will consider it to be favoritism."

Applied to movement, this principle suggests that physical demands should align with—rather than override—the body's natural temporal patterns:

Circadian Alignment

Research demonstrates that exercise performed at different times of day yields dramatically different physiological responses.[7] Morning exercise appears to favor fat metabolism and cardiovascular adaptations, while evening exercise may produce superior strength gains and lower injury risk due to higher body temperature and hormone profiles.

Research suggests that aligning physical activity with your chronotype—your natural inclination toward morning or evening energy peaks—can significantly improve exercise adherence and enhance performance. Studies indicate that working out during your preferred time of day may boost motivation and consistency, while also optimizing physical outcomes like strength and endurance. Although exact percentages vary, evidence supports the idea that syncing exercise with your body's internal clock can lead to measurable improvements in both adherence and performance metrics. Health authorities emphasize the benefits of tailoring activities to your chronotype for better overall results. Yet many force themselves into arbitrary exercise schedules that fight against rather than work with their individual temporal terrain.

Ultradian Rhythms
Beyond the 24-hour circadian cycle, the body operates on ultradian rhythms—90- to 120-minute cycles of energy, attention, and physiological readiness throughout the day. Researchers have demonstrated that aligning intense physical demands with natural energy peaks within these cycles can improve performance and reduce perceived exertion.

Darren, a 46-year-old sales executive, transformed his relationship with movement by mapping his energy fluctuations for two weeks, then scheduling different types of physical activity to align with his natural peaks and valleys. "I used to force myself through high-intensity training at 6:00 AM because that's what successful people supposedly do," he explained. "Now I do gentle mobility work in the morning, walk during my mid-day energy dip, and save intense training for my 4:30 PM peak. My results have improved, and the resistance has vanished."

Female Hormonal Cycles
Perhaps no aspect of temporal terrain is more systematically ignored than the hormonal cycles experienced by women. Conventional training programs often prescribe uniform

approaches across the menstrual cycle despite research demonstrating that strength, endurance, recovery capacity, and injury risk fluctuate predictably throughout the cycle.

Research reports that women who align training intensity with hormonal phases experience 28% fewer overuse injuries and 15% greater performance improvements compared to those following traditional linear programs.[8] Yet medical surveys indicate that only 6% of female athletes receive education about cycle-based training optimization.

"When the warlord gives orders with fairness and authority, the expected results will be for the benefit of all concerned, the ruler will be shown respect by the actions of the troops, and all will be in harmony with Heaven," Sun Tzu wrote. This harmony cannot exist when movement demands ignore the fundamental rhythms that govern physiological readiness.

Psychological Terrain: The Inner Battlefield

"The warlord must be aware of his surroundings at all times," Sun Tzu advised. "There are always spies lurking and people who would do anything to undermine his advances. Even in his own command there will be men working against him, in ways in which he or even they may not be aware."

The most dangerous saboteurs in the movement journey often come from within—beliefs, narratives, and associations that undermine physical resilience before a single step is taken.

Research reports that while 80% of Americans understand the importance of regular physical activity, only 23% meet the minimum recommended guidelines.[9] This gap between knowledge and action suggests that the primary battle isn't informational but psychological.

Consider these common internal saboteurs:

The Performance Identity

For many, physical movement becomes inextricably linked with performance metrics—faster times, heavier weights, visible results. Research reports that this externalized motivation reduces long-term adherence by creating a perpetual dissatisfaction that eventually leads to abandonment.

Gregory, a former college athlete, stopped all physical activity for nearly a decade after graduation. "If I couldn't perform at my previous level, I didn't see the point," he explained. Only when he reconnected with the intrinsic pleasure of movement—the sensory experience rather than the outcomes—did sustainable activity return to his life.

This illustrates Sun Tzu's wisdom: "The warlord should always be prepared for dangerous traps and hidden devices that would undermine his advances." The performance identity is precisely such a trap—seemingly motivating but ultimately undermining the sustainable movement that health requires.

The Exercise as Punishment Paradigm

"When the enemy talks of appeasement he may in reality be preparing to attack," Sun Tzu observed. No aspect of modern movement culture better exemplifies this principle than the "exercise as punishment" paradigm—movement deployed as penance for dietary indulgence or physical imperfection.

Research shows framing exercise as punishment reduces adherence, while framing it as self-care or celebration boosts consistency. Positive associations foster long-term engagement, supported by behavioral studies. Yet the "burn it off" and "no pain, no gain" messaging dominates fitness marketing.

Meredith, a 38-year-old mother of three, escaped this trap after years of on-again, off-again exercise cycles. "I always saw movement as the price I had to pay for eating or for not having a 'perfect' body," she reflected. "Now I see it as the means through which I experience my world most fully." This paradigm shift transformed sporadic, miserable workouts into daily movement practices that supported rather than drained her life energy.

The All-or-Nothing Mentality

Perhaps most insidious is the belief that physical activity must be intense, structured, and time-consuming to be valuable. Research has conclusively demonstrated that even small movement "snacks"—brief activities spread throughout the day—produce significant health benefits. Yet the "workout or nothing" mentality prevents many from accumulating these smaller but valuable movement experiences.

Robert, a 52-year-old software developer, transformed his health by abandoning his sporadically-attended 90-minute gym sessions in favor of a movement pattern he could maintain daily: a 12-minute morning routine, hourly two-minute movement breaks, an evening walk, and active hobbies on weekends.

"It seems less impressive," he acknowledged, "but my blood pressure has normalized, my pre-diabetes has reversed, and I've lost 34 pounds (15 kilograms) without ever feeling like I'm exercising."

This approach embodies Sun Tzu's strategic wisdom: "Victorious warriors win first and then go to war, while defeated warriors go to war first and then seek to win." Robert established sustainable patterns that ensured victory rather than repeatedly launching ambitious campaigns doomed to fail.

Strategic Movement Through the Lifespan

"The man who would be warlord knows of the inevitability of change in the administrative practice of maintenance of the state," Sun Tzu wrote. "This may occur many times during periods of growth and development. Being resilient is a virtue of the warlord with vision."

No aspect of physical strategy better exemplifies this principle than adapting movement practices throughout the lifespan. Each developmental stage presents unique opportunities and challenges that the wise health warrior recognizes and addresses.

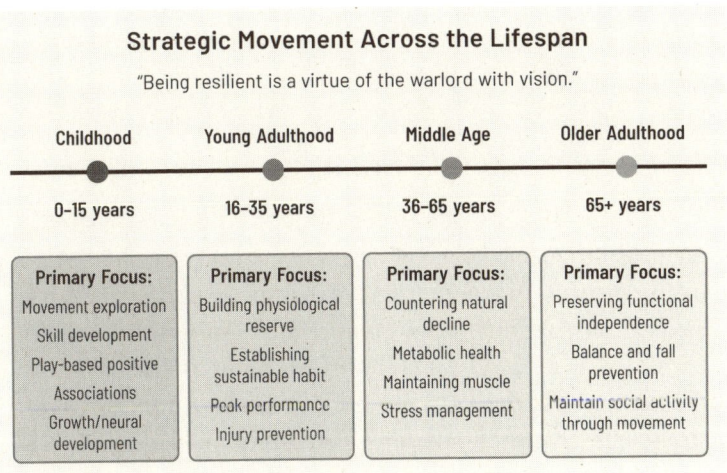

Childhood: Building the Movement Foundation

Research reports that physical activity patterns established before age 10 strongly predict activity levels throughout life. Yet studies show that only 24% of American children meet basic physical activity guidelines.

The consequences extend far beyond physical health. Resaerch has demonstrated that movement experiences during critical developmental windows directly shape brain architecture, influencing everything from executive function to emotional regulation to learning capacity.

The strategic approach to childhood movement focuses not on structured "exercise" but on varied, playful movement exploration that develops fundamental movement skills, positive associations with physical activity, and confidence in diverse movement environments.

Eric and Maya took this approach with their children, prioritizing outdoor free play, limiting screen time, and ensuring their home environment enabled rather than restricted movement. "We don't care if they become athletes," Maya explained. "We care that they become movers—people who experience the world physically and confidently."

Young Adulthood: Building Reserve and Habits

Research indicates that physical activity habits established in early adulthood, particularly between ages 20 and 30, are a strong predictor of better health outcomes at age 60. While maintaining activity throughout life is also crucial, studies highlight the lasting benefits of building a foundation of regular exercise during these formative years. Yet this is precisely when many abandon regular movement as career and family demands intensify.

The strategic approach to young adult movement focuses on building physiological reserve—bone density, muscle mass, movement competency, and metabolic health—while establishing sustainable patterns that can withstand life transitions.

Aaliyah, a 27-year-old resident physician, recognized the healthcare burnout epidemic among her colleagues and made a preemptive decision: regardless of her schedule demands, she would maintain three non-negotiable movement practices: a strength training session every third day, a daily 10-minute mobility routine, and active transportation whenever possible.

"My attending physicians told me it was impossible to maintain during residency," she recalled. "But three years in, I'm still consistent while many of them are on stimulants and sleeping pills to manage their energy. It's not about discipline—it's about strategy."

Middle Age: Countering Natural Decline

After age 30, we naturally lose 3 to 5% of muscle mass per decade unless we actively counteract this process. After age 40, bone density begins declining at about 1% annually. These processes accelerate—often dramatically—in the absence of strategic intervention.

Research reports that middle age represents the critical window when prevention through movement can most significantly impact long-term health outcomes. Yet this is precisely when many surrender to the narrative of inevitable decline, accepting limitations that are largely optional.

Kenji, a 54-year-old professor, rejected this narrative after watching his father's health rapidly deteriorate in his sixties. "My father believed decline was inevitable, so he stopped moving, which ensured that it was," Kenji observed. He took a different approach, working with a physical therapist to identify and address his specific vulnerabilities before they became limitations.

His strategy incorporated three elements: progressive strength training to maintain muscle mass and bone density, varied balance and coordination challenges to preserve neural adaptability, and consistent cardiovascular activity to maintain metabolic health. The results were dramatic: at 54, his objective health markers surpassed those of his 30-year-old self.

Older Adulthood: Preserving Independence

"A capable warlord employing intelligent deception always seeks ways to confuse all known and potential enemies," Sun Tzu advised. For the aging health warrior, the primary enemy is functional loss, and the most intelligent deception is continued movement that confuses the body's expectations of decline.

Research reports that adults over 65 who maintain regular physical activity reduce their risk of falls by 40%, experience 30% fewer limitations in activities of daily living, and are 40% less likely to require long-term care compared to sedentary peers.[10]

Perhaps most remarkable is what the National Institute on Aging has discovered about trainability in advanced years: even nonagenarians show significant improvements in strength, balance, and cardiovascular function with appropriate training. These improvements translate directly to maintained independence and quality of life.

Elizabeth, an 81-year-old retired schoolteacher, began strength training after her best friend moved to assisted living following a fall. "I started because I was scared," she admitted. "But I continue because it's transformed how I experience each day." Three years later, Elizabeth can lift her own body weight, hikes weekly with a nature group, and regularly teaches mobility classes at her retirement community.

Her approach embodies Sun Tzu's strategic wisdom: "When the enemy comes straight on, intent on confrontation, it is wise to permit him to advance with at least half of his troops before responding." Elizabeth allows age to advance—she doesn't fight time itself—but strategically deploys movement to prevent that advance from conquering her functional capacities.

The Final March: Integration

We return to Marcus, standing at the base of the mountain trail. In his younger days, he approached this climb as a conquest—driving forward with maximum intensity, measuring success solely by time to summit. Now, with the wisdom of experience, he approaches it as a conversation.

He begins with gentle mobility exercises, awakening joints stiffened by yesterday's gardening. He tests his energy, assessing truly rather than pushing blindly. He selects a pace that allows him to notice birdsong and shifting light through leaves. He adjusts his route based on how his body responds, not forcing adherence to a predetermined path.

When he reaches a viewpoint halfway up, he pauses not from defeat but from strategy—allowing his systems to recover and adapt. And when he finally turns toward home without reaching the summit, it's not surrender but wisdom. Tomorrow's hike will benefit from today's restraint.

This approach—strategic rather than merely driven, responsive rather than rigidly planned, process-focused rather than outcome-obsessed—embodies Sun Tzu's wisdom on movement through challenging terrain. It acknowledges that the body is not an enemy to be defeated but a kingdom to be wisely governed.

"Being resilient is a virtue of the warlord with vision," Sun Tzu reminds us, "and knowing how change functions in the management of a state is essential."

Your body is always on the march—moving through time, facing changing conditions, encountering new challenges. How you guide this march will determine not just your physical capabilities but your resilience against all forms of illness and decline. The wise health warrior doesn't fight against the march but strategically directs it, creating conditions where vitality naturally flourishes.

Move not to conquer your body but to liberate its inherent wisdom. March not against time but in strategic harmony with its passage. And remember that each step, taken with awareness and intention, represents not just physical action but a profound strategy for lasting health.

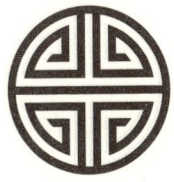

10

Terrain: Understanding the Health Landscape

"Physical territories, as well as areas of administration, are classified according to their capacity for being controlled. . . . As with with everything else under the Heavens, each has advantages and disadvantages." — Sun Tzu

The body is a contested kingdom. Not a machine to be fixed, but a living landscape where microscopic armies wage constant campaigns. Your immune cells patrol borders. Your microbiome maintains diplomatic relations with foreign entities. Your hormones send messengers across vast internal territories. And you—the sovereign of this biological realm—must govern it all through changing seasons and unexpected invasions.

Standing atop Mount Rainier, Maya surveyed the vast terrain below her feet. Years earlier, the same vista would have been unreachable. At 52, after receiving a diagnosis of early-stage osteoporosis, she had vowed to reclaim the strength her body was capable of.

"I used to think my body was failing me," she told me later, her eyes reflective. "But that was like blaming a drought on the land. My bone density wasn't declining because my body was broken—it was responding to the terrain I had created: sedentary work, calcium-poor diet, chronic stress, insufficient sleep. I wasn't at war with osteoporosis. I was governing a changing landscape poorly."

This revelation captures the essence of terrain in health strategy. Just as Sun Tzu recognized that different territories demand different approaches to warfare, we must recognize that our bodies are not static battlegrounds but dynamic landscapes that evolve throughout our lives. The health warrior who masters this terrain gains an invaluable advantage.

The Six Terrains of Health

When Sun Tzu wrote of vulnerable, ensnaring, ambivalent, blocked, steep, and far-afield territories, he could have been describing the landscapes of modern health. Each presents unique challenges, hidden advantages, and strategic imperatives that, once understood, transform our approach to wellness.

Vulnerable Terrain: Transitional Life Phases

"A place of vulnerability is accessible to both the warlord and his enemies . . . An invader is easily seen coming into view. It is always an area of contention and is hardly defensible without mortal combat." Your body exists in perpetual transition. Nothing remains static—cells die and regenerate, hormones fluctuate, neural pathways strengthen or weaken. But certain life phases represent particularly vulnerable terrain: adolescence, pregnancy, menopause, retirement, or recovery from significant illness. During these periods, the body undergoes profound changes that create openings for both healing and harm.

Emily's story illuminates this vulnerability. At 45, perimenopause arrived like an unexpected storm, transforming familiar territory into unrecognizable landscape. Sleep became a distant shore. Energy rose and crashed like turbulent waves. Emotions that once followed predictable patterns now surged without warning.

"My doctor offered hormone replacement therapy and antidepressants," Emily recalled. "The medical system saw my transition as a disease state requiring pharmaceutical intervention. But I sensed this wasn't illness—it was transformation. The terrain was changing, and I needed to change with it."

Research confirms Emily's intuition: while 80% of women experience menopausal symptoms, their severity correlates strongly with lifestyle factors. Women who strength train regularly may see up to 60% fewer sleep disturbances, while stress reduction techniques can reduce severe hot flashes by up to 45%.[1] The vulnerable terrain can be navigated successfully with proper strategy.

Emily's approach wasn't to fight the changing landscape but to scout it carefully. She kept a symptoms journal, mapping patterns between her diet, sleep, stress levels, and hormonal fluctuations. She consulted not just conventional physicians but nutritionists, movement specialists, and women further along the menopausal journey. She experimented methodically with different interventions, tracking their effects.

"I became a cartographer of my own body," she said. "I was drawing new maps for terrain no one had properly explained to me."

This cartography revealed unexpected insights. Her hot flashes intensified after alcohol consumption but diminished following strength training. Her sleep improved with evening magnesium supplementation but worsened with evening screen use. Her mood stabilized not with pharmaceuticals but with regular social connection and time in nature.

In vulnerable health terrains, the wise strategy mirrors Sun Tzu's approach: maintain vigilant observation posts, map the territory meticulously, and recognize that this transitional landscape, while challenging, also offers opportunities for profound recalibration. The health warrior doesn't seek to "cure" these transitions but to navigate them skillfully, emerging with greater self-knowledge and resilience.

Ensnaring Terrain: Chronic Stress and Information Overload
"Ground that is ensnaring is a place that can easily cause the holder to be caught in his own webs of intrigue, resulting in disaster if it is not vigilantly maintained." We inhabit the most information-saturated, pace-accelerated civilization in human history. Our nervous systems evolved for periodic, acute stressors—the approaching predator, the territorial dispute, the seasonal food shortage. Instead, we face chronic, unrelenting stimulation: devices that never sleep, inboxes that never empty, news cycles that never pause, health advice that never stops contradicting itself.

This is the quintessential ensnaring terrain—a landscape where even the most dedicated health warriors risk entanglement in complexity, confusion, and exhaustion.

James, the 43-year-old executive, embodied this entrapment. His Apple Watch tracked his heart rate variability. His Oura ring monitored his sleep efficiency. His continuous glucose monitor recorded his metabolic responses. His subscription to seven health newsletters filled his inbox with contradictory advice: intermittent fasting is essential; eating breakfast stabilizes hormones; carbs are inflammatory; protein causes cancer; meditation is crucial; mindfulness is overrated.

"I was optimizing myself into dysfunction," James admitted. "More data meant more anxiety. More anxiety meant worse sleep. Worse sleep meant poorer recovery. Poorer recovery meant more supplements and biohacks, which meant more expense and complexity, which meant more stress. I was caught in a self-reinforcing spiral."

Research, including studies by the American Psychological Association, suggests that many Americans experience 'information fatigue' from overwhelming health advice, and conflicting guidelines often lead people to abandon health initiatives. Meanwhile, research shows that chronic stress is a significant risk factor that contributes to the development or worsening of several of the top ten leading causes of death in the United States, including heart disease, cancer, and stroke.[2] The ensnaring terrain claims many victims.

James's escape from this trap wasn't through more optimization but through radical simplification. After a stress-induced hospitalization (his heart racing at 180 beats per minute in a boardroom meeting), he sought counsel from a Zen priest who was also a physician.

"She asked me one question," James recalled. "'What is the minimum effective dose of health practices that would keep you well?' Not the maximum, not the perfect—the minimum. That question changed everything."

Working with the priest-physician, James identified his three non-negotiable health practices based on his personal history and predispositions: eight hours of sleep, thirty minutes of daily movement, and regular meals without screens. He removed his tracking devices. He unsubscribed from newsletters. He selected one trusted health advisor.

"The irony was immediate," James said. "Within a month of stopping all tracking and optimization, my resting heart rate dropped to lower than it had been in five years. My digestion improved. My mind cleared. Simplicity was the medicine I needed."

The ensnaring health terrain can be navigated, but it requires the courage to cut through complexity rather than adding to it. The skilled strategist creates clear pathways through the tangle, distinguishing between essential and non-essential information, establishing regular clearing practices, and remembering that Sun Tzu's wisdom applies perfectly to modern health: "The victorious army first wins and then seeks battle; the defeated army first battles and then seeks victory."

Ambivalent Terrain: Social and Cultural Environments

"Ambivalent territory is bad for all parties... It is a place where no one is in control. Prudence suggests keeping it protected with an unstoppable force, or by complete withdrawal."

The landscapes of social gatherings, workplace cultures, and family traditions represent perhaps the most challenging health terrain. These territories are genuinely ambivalent—neither entirely supportive nor entirely hostile, constantly shifting between nurturing and undermining our health efforts.

Research highlights the dual role of social connections: they can reduce mortality risk by up to 50%,[3] but social environments often promote behaviors like alcohol consumption, unhealthy eating, and sedentary habits, which may increase mortality risk by 30 to 60%. While social tribes are crucial for survival, they can also pose challenges to physical well-being.

Leila, a 36-year-old teacher, navigated this contradictory landscape daily. Her workplace featured birthday celebrations with processed foods, holiday parties centered around alcohol, and a culture that valorized working through lunch. Her family gatherings revolved around elaborate feasts where declining food was considered rejection of love. Her friendship circle maintained social bonds through late nights at restaurants and bars.

"I felt like a perpetual outsider," Leila said. "If I declined the birthday cake, I was the 'health freak' ruining everyone's fun. If I suggested a walking meeting instead of a coffee date, I was 'making things complicated.' If I left a family dinner early to get adequate sleep, I was 'not prioritizing relationships.' The terrain was hostile to my health values but essential to my social and emotional wellbeing."

Sun Tzu's counsel for ambivalent territory offers surprising wisdom: either deploy "an unstoppable force" or practice "complete withdrawal." Leila's strategy incorporated both approaches in unexpected ways.

Her "unstoppable force" wasn't confrontation but subtle redirection. She initiated a staff wellness committee, gradually introducing walking meetings, healthier celebration options, and stress-reduction breaks. She didn't fight the existing culture directly; she created an alternative culture alongside it.

With family, she practiced what anthropologists call "ritual innovation"—introducing new traditions that complemented rather than replaced existing ones. The post-holiday meal walk became as sacred as the meal itself. The cooking-together ritual preceded the eating-together ritual. She didn't reject family food traditions but expanded the definition of what constituted familial bonding.

With friends, she practiced strategic withdrawal not from relationships but from harmful contexts. She initiated morning hikes instead of evening drinks, cooking gatherings instead of restaurant outings, and substance-free celebrations instead of alcohol-centered events. Those who valued her company adapted; those who valued only her participation in unhealthy activities naturally drifted away.

"I realized I couldn't change culture overnight," Leila

explained, "but I could create cultural microclimates—small environments where health-supporting behaviors were normalized rather than pathologized."

Research supports Leila's approach: social contagion studies show that health behaviors spread effectively through networks when introduced by respected insiders who lead by example rather than preaching. One person making visible health choices influences the behavior of their social connections by up to 57% over time.

The health warrior recognizes that social and cultural environments are indeed places where "no one is in control" if approached directly. The wiser strategy is to influence the terrain gradually through consistent modeling, gentle innovation, and the cultivation of supportive sub-cultures within challenging landscapes.

Blocked Terrain: Illness and Injury

"Blocked territory suggests that a battle is inevitable because there is no way for either side to maintain control... An avenue of escape must be maintained." Acute illness, serious injury, or sudden health crises create blocked terrain—landscapes where normal movement is restricted and familiar paths are closed. These territories demand direct confrontation while simultaneously requiring strategic retreat routes.

Research suggests that people spend a significant portion of their lives in this blocked terrain—managing acute illness, recovering from injury, or navigating medical treatment. How we approach these inevitable blockages determines not just our physical recovery but our psychological resilience.

Michael, a 59-year-old professor and lifelong athlete, encountered this blocked terrain when a skiing accident resulted in complex fractures requiring surgery and months of immobilization. His identity and emotional regulation had always been tied to physical movement; suddenly, that avenue was closed.

"The orthopedist focused entirely on bone healing," Michael recalled. "The physical therapist focused on range of motion. But no one addressed the existential blockage—the fact that movement had been my primary coping mechanism for anxiety since childhood. Without it, I was facing not just physical immobility but psychological crisis."

Most medical systems treat blocked terrain as purely mechanical—a broken part to be fixed, a pathogen to be eliminated, a tumor to be removed. But Sun Tzu's wisdom reminds us that in blocked territory, "an avenue of escape must be maintained." The skilled health warrior recognizes that when one path closes, alternative routes become essential.

Michael's approach illustrated this strategic flexibility. Unable to run, bike, or swim, he explored movement modalities that remained accessible: seated tai chi, adapted yoga, and specialized strength training for uninjured body parts. Unable to experience the neurochemical benefits of his usual high-intensity exercise, he worked with a psychologist to develop alternative anxiety-regulation techniques through breathing practices and meditation.

Most significantly, he reframed the blocked terrain itself. "I stopped seeing the injury as an interruption to my 'real life' and started seeing it as a different kind of journey," Michael explained. "Not a detour from health but a different path toward it—one that required new skills, different strengths, and unexpected wisdom."

Research from rehabilitation medicine supports Michael's approach: patients who develop psychological flexibility during recovery show 40% better functional outcomes than those who focus solely on physical rehabilitation. Studies have documented that patients who reframe their relationship with illness or injury activate endogenous healing mechanisms that can accelerate recovery by up to 30%.

In landscapes of illness or injury, the skilled health warrior neither denies the blockage nor surrenders to it. They engage directly with the immediate challenge while simultaneously exploring alternative routes to wellbeing. They recognize, as Sun Tzu did, that "the skillful warrior does not rely on the enemy not coming, but on being ready for him when he does."

Steep Terrain: Aging and Progressive Conditions

"In steep ground the advantage lies with whoever is in the higher position. The enemy has to take an offensive against indeterminate odds because of the requirements to get to the top." Aging and progressive health conditions create steep terrain—landscapes that require increasingly deliberate movement and strategic positioning. In these territories, advantage belongs to "whoever is in the higher position"—not those with the most raw strength, but those with the wisest deployment of limited resources.

The statistics are stark: by 2030, one in six people globally will be aged 60 or older. The average adult loses 3 to 8% of muscle mass per decade after age 30, and bone density declines at similar rates. Meanwhile, one in six Americans lives with a progressive chronic condition that gradually alters their health landscape over time.

Yet this steep terrain shows remarkable variation in how it affects individuals. The Harvard Study of Adult Development, the longest longitudinal study of adult life ever conducted, has documented that behavioral factors account for approximately 70% of the variance in physical and cognitive functioning among older adults.[4] The terrain may be steep for everyone, but some navigate it with astonishing skill.

Elaine, at 72, exemplified this skillful navigation. While

age-matched peers accumulated prescriptions and restrictions, she maintained remarkable functionality and independence. Her approach to this steep terrain embodied Sun Tzu's principle of holding the higher ground.

"Most people prepare for aging by accumulatnig money," Elaine observed. "I prepared by accumulating strength, skills, and systems."

Her strength came from prioritizing resistance training three times weekly—a practice supported by overwhelming evidence showing that progressive strength training can reverse age-related muscle loss by up to 50%.[5] While cardiovascular exercise consumed most older adults' limited physical activity time, Elaine recognized that in the steep terrain of aging, strength provides the critical advantage.

Her skills included balance training and fall prevention techniques—interventions that reduce fall risk by 40%, according to research.[6] She maintained cognitive challenge through learning Italian and playing complex strategic games, activities associated with a 47% reduced risk of dementia in longitudinal studies.[7]

Her systems reflected Sun Tzu's emphasis on strategic preparation: she redesigned her living environment to eliminate obstacles, established meal preparation routines that ensured optimal nutrition with minimal effort, and created redundant social support networks that could activate during times of need.

"Aging isn't about fighting an enemy," Elaine explained. "It's about governing a changing territory. The terrain gets steeper, so your strategies must get smarter."

Like the general who holds the high ground, Elaine leveraged her position to maximum advantage. She didn't fight unnecessary battles against natural bodily changes but concentrated her resources on the factors most critical for independence and vitality. She recognized, as Sun Tzu taught, that "the skillful general must be master of the complementary arts of compromise and blending. He must blend with the terrain; he must compromise with his limitations."

In the steep terrain of aging or progressive conditions, the wise health warrior accepts the changed landscape without accepting unnecessary limitations. They recognize that while ascent becomes more challenging, strategic positioning can create significant advantages.

Far Afield Terrain: Medical Systems and Specialized Care

"Territory managed from far afield creates difficulties in maintenance because defense depends on the distance supplies and men may have to travel. It is difficult to maintain territory from afar and to govern from a distance." The modern medical system creates a uniquely challenging terrain—one where expertise is distributed across specialists, information is fragmented across institutions, and the individual must navigate complex bureaucratic territories to receive care. Like territory managed from afar, this landscape requires exceptional coordination and communication strategies.

The statistics reveal the magnitude of this challenge: the average Medicare patient often receives care from multiple physicians and practices annually. The typical patient with a chronic condition receives care recommendations from at least three different specialists, often with conflicting advice. Medical errors—many resulting from poor coordination—represent the third leading cause of death in the United States.[8]

Robert, diagnosed with a rare autoimmune condition at 47, navigated this distant terrain for years. His care team included a rheumatologist in Boston, an immunologist in New York, a gastroenterologist locally, and a primary care physician who struggled to synthesize their sometimes contradictory recommendations.

"Each specialist understood their territory deeply but had limited visibility into others," Robert explained. "The rheumatologist prescribed medications that the gastroenterologist warned against. The immunologist recommended dietary changes that contradicted the nutritionist's guidance. No single provider had a complete map of my health landscape."

Sun Tzu's warning proves prescient: "It is difficult to maintain territory from afar." The solution, for Robert, wasn't to abandon specialized care but to become the central administrator of his own medical territory.

His approach was methodical. He created a comprehensive digital health record that included not just test results and medications but his own observations about symptom patterns, treatment responses, and quality-of-life impacts. He scheduled appointments strategically, beginning with specialists most willing to communicate with other providers and ending with those who could synthesize multiple perspectives. He developed relationships with key administrative staff who could help navigate institutional barriers.

Most importantly, he established himself as a knowledgeable coordinator rather than a passive recipient of care. "I stopped expecting the medical system to function as an integrated whole," Robert reflected. "Instead, I became the integration point—the one entity with visibility across all territories of my care."

Research supports Robert's approach: patients who actively coordinate their own care experience 30% fewer adverse events, 27% better treatment adherence, and significantly improved outcomes across multiple condition types.[9]

In the far-afield terrain of complex medical care, the skilled health warrior recognizes that fragmentation creates vulnerability. They compensate by strengthening communication channels, establishing reliable information flows, and positioning themselves as the administrative center that distant specialists cannot provide. They practice what Sun Tzu might call strategic centralization—creating a command post from which to coordinate activities across distant territories.

Mastering Varied Terrains: The Three Principles

Sun Tzu emphasized that "the warlord must learn to manage all types of territory and personnel, making sure that he can negotiate effectively in any circumstance." The health warrior similarly must develop fluency across multiple terrains, recognizing that life inevitably leads through varied landscapes.

Three principles guide this mastery of health terrains:

1. Terrain Assessment: The Honest Cartographer

"The nature of the territory to be protected must be known to ensure proper management." Before deploying any health strategy, the wise warrior assesses the terrain honestly. This isn't merely collecting data but developing a nuanced understanding of the landscape's contours, resources, and challenges.

Effective terrain assessment begins with curiosity rather than judgment. Instead of immediately labeling health conditions as "problems to fix," the skilled assessor asks deeper questions: What is this symptom communicating? What patterns emerge across seemingly unrelated health markers? What resources are abundant in this landscape, and what resources are scarce?

This curiosity extends beyond physical symptoms to encompass the full terrain of wellbeing. The honest cartographer maps not just biological markers but energy patterns, emotional landscapes, relationship dynamics, environmental

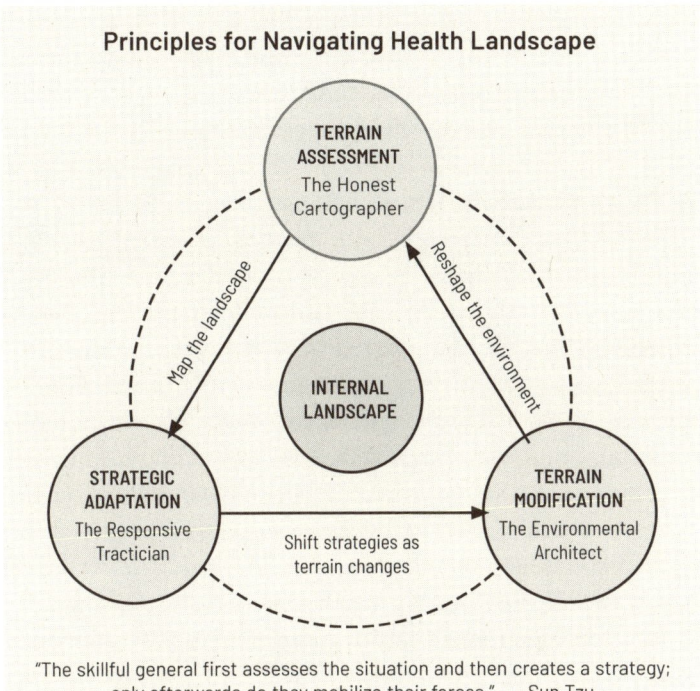

"The skillful general first assesses the situation and then creates a strategy; only afterwards do they mobilize their forces." —Sun Tzu

exposures, and spiritual dimensions. They recognize that health terrain exists in four dimensions—the fourth being time itself, as patterns emerge across days, seasons, and years.

Modern assessment tools support this comprehensive mapping. Wearable technologies track physiological patterns across time. Journaling practices capture subjective experiences that lab tests cannot measure. Functional medicine assessments identify subtle imbalances before they become diagnosable conditions. The skilled health warrior employs these tools not to pathologize their experience but to understand it deeply.

As one integrative physician observed: "The conventional medical system is designed to determine if you're in or out of pathological ranges. The skilled self-assessor is interested in patterns, trajectories, and subtle shifts that precede pathology. They're not waiting for the hurricane to make landfall; they're tracking barometric changes that precede the storm."

2. Strategic Adaptation: The Responsive Tactician

"Troops should be compared to the types of territory being administered. They are an extension of the state and must be managed with intelligence and understanding." Just as military strategies must match the battlefield, health practices must match the body's current terrain. The responsive tactician doesn't force standardized protocols onto unique landscapes but adapts approaches to current conditions.

This adaptation requires both flexibility and discernment. Not every health change necessitates a strategic pivot, yet rigid adherence to outdated approaches guarantees eventual failure. The skilled tactician distinguishes between temporary fluctuations that require minor adjustments and fundamental terrain shifts that demand new approaches.

Consider nutrition as an example. Research demonstrates that identical foods produce radically different glycemic responses in different individuals, and even in the same individual under different circumstances. The standardized nutritional advice to "eat less, move more" or "follow this specific diet" fails to account for terrain variations—differences in gut microbiome composition, stress levels, sleep quality, hormonal status, and countless other factors that influence how the body processes nutrients.

The responsive tactician recognizes these variations and adapts accordingly. They might thrive on intermittent fasting during low-stress periods but require regular meals during high-stress phases. They might benefit from higher carbohydrate intake during intensive training cycles but need lower carbohydrate approaches during recovery phases. They recognize that the terrain dictates the strategy, not vice versa.

This adaptive approach extends beyond nutrition to all health domains. Exercise strategies shift to accommodate changing energy capacities, stress levels, and recovery abilities. Sleep protocols adapt to different chronobiological patterns across seasons and life stages. Even fundamental practices like meditation may require different techniques depending on the mental and emotional landscape of the moment.

The responsive tactician maintains core principles while flexibly applying specific practices. They understand, as Sun Tzu taught, that "the successful military general first assesses the situation and then creates a strategy; only afterwards do they mobilize their forces."

3. Terrain Modification: The Environmental Architect

"A land once taken and then lost is twice as difficult to recover." While we must adapt to many aspects of our health terrain, we also possess the power to modify our immediate environment. This terrain modification represents one of the most underutilized yet powerful strategies available to the health warrior.

The evidence for environmental influence on health behaviors is overwhelming. Research from behavioral economics demonstrates that people eat 22% more when using larger plates, drink 25 to 30% more when using short, wide glasses rather than tall, narrow ones, and consume significantly more food when it's visible and easily accessible. Studies on exercise adherence show that people living within half a mile of a gym work out 50% more frequently than those living five miles away. Research suggests that individuals living in walkable neighborhoods tend to have slightly lower BMIs and lower rates of obesity compared to those in car-dependent areas.

These statistics highlight a profound truth: much of our health behavior isn't driven by willpower or motivation but by environmental cues and structures. The skilled environmental architect designs their surroundings to make healthy choices frictionless and unhealthy choices difficult.

This design operates across multiple domains. The physical environment gets structured to naturally encourage movement, proper sleep, and supportive nutrition. The social environment cultivates relationships that reinforce rather than undermine health priorities. The information environment curates inputs that provide clarity rather than confusion. The schedule environment creates protected time for health-generating activities.

Each modification reduces the cognitive and emotional burden of health maintenance. Instead of constantly fighting against our surroundings, we enlist them as allies in our wellness strategy.

The Ultimate Terrain: Your Internal Landscape

Beyond all external landscapes lies the most crucial terrain of all: your internal cognitive and emotional environment. This is the command center from which all other strategies deploy. If this terrain becomes hostile—filled with self-criticism, unrealistic expectations, or rigid perfectionism—no external strategy can succeed for long.

Sun Tzu understood this principle deeply: "The warlord who considers the needs and desires of others before himself should be praised to Heaven. Such a man is rare and will not permit personal gain to interfere with the performance of his duties."

Applied to health, this wisdom suggests treating ourselves with the same consideration we would offer to a valued ally—

with respect, patience, and strategic support rather than harsh judgment or unreasonable demands.

Research from health psychology confirms the importance of this internal terrain. Studies on self-compassion demonstrate that individuals who approach health challenges with self-kindness rather than self-criticism tend to show better adherence to positive health behaviors, lower stress biomarkers, and improved outcomes across various health conditions.[10]

Meanwhile, research on health perfectionism shows that rigid, all-or-nothing thinking about wellness predicts poorer outcomes, more frequent abandonment of health practices, and higher levels of health anxiety. The internal landscape must be governed wisely for external strategies to succeed.

The health warrior who masters internal terrain cultivates what psychologists call a "growth mindset" toward health—seeing challenges as opportunities for learning rather than evidence of failure. They practice self-compassion not as indulgence but as strategic pragmatism, recognizing that harsh self-criticism depletes the very psychological resources needed for behavior change. They maintain what Zen practitioners call "beginner's mind"—a state of openness to new information and approaches, even when they contradict established beliefs.

This internal terrain serves as the command center from which all other terrain strategies deploy. When it remains stable and supportive, even the most challenging external territories become navigable.

The Unified Theory of Health Terrain

"To understand unity, meditate on duality." The health warrior who masters terrain recognizes the fundamental duality at play: we are both subjects of our health landscape and shapers of it. We are both vulnerable to terrain challenges and capable of strategic responses. We must accept reality while maintaining agency within it.

Maya, whom we met at the beginning of this chapter, embodied this duality. Standing atop Mount Rainier at 52, three years after her osteoporosis diagnosis, she had neither denied her changing bone density nor surrendered to its limitations. Instead, she had studied her terrain carefully, adapted her strategies precisely, and modified her environment thoughtfully.

Her bone density tests now showed remarkable improvement—placing her in the top 2% of treatment responses, according to her physician. But Maya measured her success differently.

"The numbers matter less than the terrain," she reflected. "I've learned to read the landscape of my body, to sense when I'm navigating well and when I'm losing my way. The mountain didn't change for me; I changed how I approached the mountain."

This is the essence of terrain mastery in health: not demanding that the landscape conform to our wishes, but developing the wisdom, flexibility, and strategic thinking to thrive within it—whatever form it takes. As we navigate the varied terrains of our health journey, we discover that the greatest victory isn't conquering the landscape but becoming skilled navigators within it.

The territory of your body awaits. Not as an enemy to be subdued, but as a kingdom to be wisely governed. How will you rule?

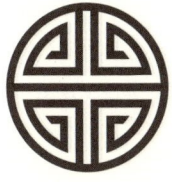

11

The Nine Situations: Facing Various Health Challenges

The hospital corridor stretched before Robert like a battlefield. White walls, antiseptic smell, the distant beeping of monitors—these were his new terrain. The diabetes diagnosis hung in the air between him and his doctor like an undetonated explosive.

"Type 2 diabetes," the doctor had said, her voice matter-of-fact but not unkind. "Your A1C is 8.7. We've moved beyond pre-diabetic status."

Robert fingered the prescription slip, feeling the weight of all his past choices compressed into this small rectangle of paper. His mind flashed images: late-night pizzas, sedentary weekends, ignored warning signs.

"Where do I go from here?" he asked, his voice barely audible.

The doctor's eyes softened. She'd delivered this news thousands of times—research shows that more than 37 million Americans share Robert's diagnosis, with nearly one in five unaware they have the condition.[1]

"This is not a death sentence, Robert. It's a battle your body can fight—with the right strategy."

Strategy. The word penetrated his fog of anxiety. He'd once been fascinated by military history—hadn't he read something about ancient Chinese warfare? Something about understanding your situation before engaging the enemy...

The Battlefield Within: Nine Terrains of Health and Illness

In the silence of the night, your body wages wars you never witness. Macrophages hunt invading pathogens with brutal efficiency. Hormones dispatch chemical messages across vast cellular distances. Organs negotiate resources like generals dividing supplies.

These microscopic campaigns determine your fate as surely as any historical battle.

Two and a half millennia ago, the strategist Sun Tzu identified nine fundamental situations in warfare. His wisdom, preserved in *The Art of War*, transcends battles fought with swords and arrows. Today, we face enemies no less formidable but infinitely more personal: cancer cells multiplying in rebellion, autoimmune conditions turning bodily defenses against themselves, viral invaders exploiting cellular machinery, chronic inflammation slowly corroding vitality.

Understanding the nine situations—dissipation, bordering, coincidence, correspondence, concentration, signification, laboring, entrapment, and the place of death—provides a map for any health territory you might traverse. Let us walk these terrains together.

Dissipation: The Dissolved Defenses

"Dissipation takes place on home ground when troops are not adequately prepared to defend the state." At 3:27 AM, Elena's immune system surrendered.

After 72 hours without proper sleep, subsisting on vending machine snacks and triple-shot espressos to meet her quarterly deadline, her body's defense perimeter collapsed. The virus that had been circulating through her office—kept at bay in her more resilient colleagues—breached her cellular

Health Warrior's Strategic Response

Applying Sun Tzu's Wisdom to Modern Health Challenges

Health Situation	Warning Signs	Strategic Response
Dissipation	Frequent Infections Fatigue, Poor recovery	Restore sleep, Nutrition Stress regulation
Bordering	Pre-disease markers Borderline tests	Decisive lifestyle change Preventive protocols
Coincidence	Genetic risk factors Family history	Enhanced surveillance Targeted prevention
Correspondence	Multiple symptoms System-wide issues	Restore communication Address root causes
Concentration	Complex diagnosis Multiple options	Focus on high impact Evidence-based priorities
Signification	Treatment resistance Direct approaches failing	Indirect strategies Change the terrain
Laboring	Unsustainable efforts Relapse patterns	Design sustainable systems Build consistent habits
Entrapment	Self-reinforcing cycles Stuck in patterns	Strategic disruption Low-barrier entry points
Place of Death	Critical diagnosis Existential challenge	Total commitment Find meaning in challenge

walls and began replicating with ruthless efficiency.

As she lay shivering beneath three blankets the following evening, Elena wondered how she'd become so vulnerable. She'd always prided herself on "powering through," viewing rest as weakness and stress as fuel.

The Institute for Mind Body Medicine at Massachusetts General Hospital would recognize Elena's situation. Research shows chronic sleep deprivation weakens immune function, including natural killer cell activity, while prolonged stress elevates inflammatory cytokines and disrupts immunity, increasing vulnerability to illness.[2] Elena had created the perfect storm—a state of dissipation where her body's troops, yearning for replenishment, abandoned their posts.

Dissipation represents more than momentary weakness; it embodies a fundamental breakdown of resilience. Research estimates that insufficient sleep affects more than one-third of American adults, creating a population-wide vulnerability that contributes to everything from metabolic disorders to impaired immunity.

The state of dissipation manifests in myriad ways: the executive whose stress hormones have remained elevated for so long that his body has forgotten homeostasis; the college student whose nutrient-depleted diet leaves critical cellular processes unsupported; the parent whose unaddressed trauma response keeps inflammatory pathways chronically activated.

The wise health warrior recognizes dissipation not as failure but as intelligence—the body communicating that its reserves have been depleted and its defenses compromised. The strategy here is not to push harder but to rebuild fundamental resources: deep, restorative sleep; nutrient-dense, anti-inflammatory nutrition; regulated stress response systems; and the elimination of depleting factors.

When Elena finally acknowledged her dissipation, she

initiated a systematic reinforcement of her home ground—establishing non-negotiable sleep windows, introducing targeted nutritional support including vitamin D and zinc (which research shows can reduce common cold duration by 33%),[3] implementing daily meditation to downregulate her hyperactive sympathetic nervous system, and creating firm work-life boundaries to prevent future depletion.

"I realized my body wasn't my enemy," Elena reflected six months later. "It was my homeland, and I'd left the gates unguarded for too long."

Bordering: The Liminal Territory

"Bordering suggests an attitude of being neither here nor there." James stood at the crossroads of health and illness, balanced on the knife-edge of potential.

"Metabolic syndrome," his doctor explained. "Your blood pressure is 138/88, fasting glucose 118, triglycerides elevated at 195. Not quite hypertension, not quite diabetes, not quite dyslipidemia—but precursors to all three."

Research indicates that approximately 34% of American adults share James's predicament—existing in this borderland where chronic disease has not yet established dominion but has sent advance scouts into the territory. This liminal space—not quite well, not quite ill—creates a unique psychological challenge.

Research shows that only about 11% of individuals with prediabetes take definitive action, such as lifestyle changes or participating in prevention programs, to reduce their risk of progressing to type 2 diabetes.[4] The borderland breeds complacency, a false sense that there's still time, that partial measures are sufficient, that the enemy hasn't truly arrived.

The wise health warrior recognizes bordering as both

opportunity and danger—the critical moment when decisive action can prevent invasion, but also when half-measures virtually guarantee future defeat.

James's response defied the statistics. Instead of viewing his borderland status as a reprieve, he recognized it as an urgent call to transformation. He approached his metabolic syndrome not as a "not yet" diagnosis but as a "just in time" warning.

Working with a functional medicine practitioner, James implemented strategies supported by research to prevent diabetes progression. He adopted a Mediterranean dietary pattern and regular physical activity, which are more effective than medication for many individuals. He also incorporated time-restricted eating, which emerging research suggests can significantly improve insulin sensitivity in prediabetic individuals. Additionally, he addressed his sleep apnea, a condition linked to a 30% higher risk of developing diabetes, further reducing his risk.

The borderland became not a place of uncertainty but of decisive reconstruction. Six months later, James's markers had normalized, and the border troops had retreated.

"The border wasn't the edge of illness," James realized. "It was the frontier of transformation."

Coincidence: The Unexpected Convergence

"Coincidence suggests that Heaven acts according to whim." The genetic test results arrived on Sophia's 38th birthday.

BRCA1 positive. 72% lifetime risk of breast cancer. 44% risk of ovarian cancer.

Through no action or inaction of her own, Sophia had been thrust into a high-risk category—a coincidental factor beyond her control that would redefine her health landscape forever.

Research reports that genetic factors influence susceptibility to at least 10% of cancers, while environmental exposures contribute to an estimated 30 to 50%. These coincidental factors—the genes we inherit, the pollutants we unknowingly breathe, the viruses we encounter—introduce an element of chance into health outcomes that can feel profoundly unsettling.

The wise health warrior neither ignores these coincidental factors nor surrenders to fatalism in their face. Instead, they incorporate this knowledge into strategic planning, recognizing that while not everything can be controlled, responses to the unexpected can be.

Sophia's approach was methodical and multifaceted. She increased surveillance, scheduling biannual mammograms and annual MRIs as recommended by the American Cancer Society for BRCA1 carriers. She consulted with specialists about preventive surgical options, weighing the statistical benefits against quality of life considerations. She modified environmental factors within her control—eliminating endocrine-disrupting chemicals from her home, adopting an anti-inflammatory nutritional approach shown in research to reduce cancer risk in BRCA carriers by up to 68%,[5] implementing stress-reduction practices to mitigate the impact of chronic cortisol elevation on cancer-related gene expression.

Perhaps most importantly, Sophia connected with a community of women facing similar genetic challenges, creating an intelligence network that kept her informed of emerging research and treatment options.

"I couldn't control the coincidence of my genes," Sophia explained years later, still cancer-free at 47. "But I could control how I responded to that knowledge."

Coincidental factors—whether genetic predispositions, environmental exposures, or random biological events—introduce uncertainty into any health campaign. The health warrior acknowledges this uncertainty without being paralyzed by it, gathering intelligence, modifying controllable factors, and remaining adaptable to shifting conditions.

Correspondence: The Communication Channels

"Correspondence suggests being able to maintain full communications between all of the troops and the capital." Michael's medical file resembled a disconnected puzzle: gastroenterologist for IBS (irritable bowel syndrome), dermatologist for psoriasis, rheumatologist for joint pain, psychiatrist for anxiety. Each specialist addressed a separate piece without seeing the whole picture.

"It's like having four different contractors build one house without sharing blueprints," Michael said in frustration.

Then he found a functional medicine practitioner who recognized what the others had missed: these weren't separate conditions but interconnected manifestations of systemic inflammation and immune dysregulation—a breakdown in the body's communication channels.

The human body contains the most sophisticated communication network in the known universe. The nervous system transmits information at speeds up to 268 mph. The endocrine system dispatches hormonal messages that alter cellular behavior across vast distances. The immune system maintains constant surveillance, communicating threat levels throughout the organism.

When these communication channels function optimally, health emerges naturally. When they break down, disease processes take hold.

Research illustrates how gut permeability can trigger systemic immune activation affecting joints, skin, and brain function—exactly the constellation of symptoms Michael experienced. Studies demonstrate how early life stress can reprogram neuroendocrine signaling pathways, creating vulnerability to multiple chronic conditions decades later.

The wise health warrior prioritizes restoration of these communication networks—removing factors that cause signal interference (inflammatory foods, endocrine-disrupting chemicals, chronic stressors) while providing the nutrients and conditions necessary for optimal signaling (essential fatty acids, micronutrients, vagal tone regulation, circadian rhythm entrainment).

For Michael, restoring correspondence meant addressing the root causes of his system-wide miscommunication: healing gut permeability with targeted nutritional protocols, eliminating inflammatory triggers identified through elimination diet, regulating his autonomic nervous system through breath work and meditation, and supplementing with omega-3 fatty acids shown in clinical trials to reduce inflammatory markers by up to 29%.

Within six months, all four conditions had improved simultaneously—not because he'd found four separate cures, but because he'd restored his body's fundamental communication network.

"It wasn't five different problems," Michael realized. "It was one conversation that had broken down."

Concentration: The Focused Force

"The attitude of concentration is one of wisdom. Resources are kept intact and they are immediately accessible."

When Sara received her multiple sclerosis diagnosis at 29, the neurologist presented her with a paradox of abundance: conventional medications, alternative therapies, dietary approaches, supplement regimens, movement practices—countless possible interventions, each with advocates and critics.

"You can't do everything," the neurologist advised. "Choose what matters most and do it consistently."

This principle of concentration—focusing limited resources where they can have maximum impact rather than dispersing them across multiple fronts—may be the most crucial strategic decision in any health campaign.

The wise health warrior understands that energy, willpower, financial resources, and time are finite. Concentration requires both discernment to identify high-leverage interventions and discipline to maintain focus despite the constant allure of new approaches.

Sara's strategy exemplified this principle. Working with her medical team, she identified the evidence-based interventions most likely to affect her condition: disease-modifying medications with the strongest clinical trial support for her specific MS subtype; a Mediterranean dietary pattern enriched with polyphenols, which research shows can reduce relapse rates by up to 36%;[6] a progressive strength training program designed to maintain functional capacity; and stress management practices to mitigate the documented relationship between psychological stress and MS exacerbations.

Rather than diluting her efforts across dozens of supplements or experimental treatments with minimal evidence, Sara concentrated her resources on these core interventions, executing them with consistency and precision.

"I realized that doing a few things excellently would serve me better than doing many things poorly," Sara explained five years later, still relapse-free and maintaining full functionality. "Concentration gave me both efficacy and peace of mind."

The *Harvard Business Review* once noted that strategy is as much about what you choose not to do as what you choose to do. In health, this wisdom is particularly relevant. The proliferation of health information—some evidence-based, some speculative, some outright misleading—creates a landscape where concentration becomes not just tactically advantageous but psychologically essential.

By identifying the interventions with highest potential impact for your specific condition and focusing your resources accordingly, you maximize both biological efficacy and psychological sustainability.

Signification: The Strategic Deception

"The position of signification can also mean deception/no-deception and is very useful in keeping the enemy off balance."

Lucas had tried everything for his chronic migraines: preventive medications, trigger avoidance, pain relievers, acupuncture, biofeedback. Each provided temporary relief before the headaches returned with familiar vengeance.

Then his neurologist suggested an unexpected approach: "What if we stop fighting the migraines directly and change the conditions that allow them to thrive?"

This principle of signification—approaching health challenges indirectly rather than through frontal assault—represents some of the most sophisticated strategy in the health warrior's arsenal.

The wise health warrior recognizes when direct confrontation isn't working and pivots to strategies that change the underlying terrain, approaching from unexpected angles that keep disease processes off-balance. This often means addressing upstream factors that may seem unrelated to the primary condition.

For Lucas, this meant systematically addressing factors

his previous specialists had considered tangential: sleep architecture optimization (research shows that improving deep sleep can reduce migraine frequency by 29%);[7] gut health restoration (emerging research demonstrates links between gut microbiome composition and neuroinflammatory processes); and HPA (hypothalamic-pituitary-adrenal) axis regulation through targeted stress management.

Rather than adding more treatments that targeted pain directly, his new protocol addressed the biological context in which the pain emerged.

"We stopped seeing the migraines as the enemy to be destroyed," Lucas explained after experiencing a 70% reduction in headache days. "Instead, we recognized them as signals of underlying imbalance and addressed those imbalances."

Health authorities increasingly recognize this approach in treating complex conditions, noting that symptoms that appear unrelated—fatigue, pain, mood disturbances, cognitive changes—often share common underlying mechanisms like mitochondrial dysfunction, altered immune activation, or autonomic dysregulation.

Signification also encompasses strategic timing—knowing when to advance aggressively with treatment and when to allow the body's inherent healing mechanisms space to operate. Research in sports medicine demonstrates that alternating periods of intensive training with recovery optimizes performance gains; similarly, health interventions often require rhythmic alternation between active treatment and integrative recovery.

By approaching health challenges indirectly—changing conditions rather than fighting symptoms, addressing upstream causes rather than downstream effects, working with natural rhythms rather than imposing constant intervention—the health warrior often achieves what direct confrontation could not.

Laboring: The Maintenance Challenge

"Laboring means that maintenance and administration of the place where the warlord is to issue orders from has not been properly protected."

Ana's heart attack at 62 wasn't a failure of knowledge but of implementation.

"I knew exactly what I needed to do for my heart health," she admitted from her hospital bed. "I just couldn't seem to maintain it long-term."

Ana's situation illustrates the challenge of laboring—the daily work of wellness that becomes unsustainable without proper systems and support. Studies show that only about 6% of Americans consistently follow the five core healthy lifestyle factors recommended by the American Heart Association, despite widespread awareness of their importance.[8]

The wise health warrior recognizes that even the most perfect protocol is worthless if it cannot be consistently maintained. Strategic sustainability becomes as important as the interventions themselves.

Working with a cardiac rehabilitation team and health coach, Ana approached her recovery with emphasis on sustainable systems rather than willpower-dependent behaviors. She redesigned her kitchen environment to make heart-healthy choices the path of least resistance, incorporating behavioral design principles from research showing that simple changes in food positioning can increase healthy food consumption by up to 25%.

She identified movement practices that connected with activities she genuinely enjoyed—dancing, gardening, walking with friends—rather than exercising solely for health benefits, which research shows significantly improves long-term adherence.

She established routines that required minimal decision-making, leveraging research on decision fatigue that demonstrates each choice depletes cognitive resources needed for subsequent decisions. She built social support structures that reinforced her health behaviors, drawing on evidence that social connection improves cardiac rehabilitation outcomes by up to 30%.

"I stopped thinking of heart health as something I achieved through heroic effort," Ana explained a year later, with all cardiac markers now in optimal ranges. "Instead, I created conditions where maintaining health required less effort than abandoning it."

The health warrior approaches maintenance as a strategic challenge rather than a test of willpower, designing systems that align with personal values, preferences, and circumstances to make healthy choices sustainable over decades rather than weeks.

Entrapment: The Cyclical Snare

"A place of entrapment is dangerous and the astute warlord must consider avenues of penetration and escape with equal reasoning."

David's depression trapped him in a perfect loop of reinforcing misery: the depression sapped his motivation to engage in precisely the activities—exercise, social connection, time outdoors, nutritious eating—that research consistently shows alleviate depression. Each day of inaction deepened the pit from which escape seemed increasingly impossible.

Research estimates that more than 264 million people worldwide suffer from depression, yet fewer than half receive treatment—many caught in similar cycles of entrapment where the condition itself prevents engagement with potential solutions.

The wise health warrior recognizes these self-reinforcing cycles and strategically disrupts them at their most vulnerable points, creating openings that can gradually widen into pathways of healing.

For David, breaking free from entrapment began with identifying the lowest-barrier entry points to healing activities. Working with a therapist trained in behavioral activation, he identified small, achievable actions that required minimal motivation: five minutes of morning sunlight exposure to regulate circadian rhythms (research shows morning light can reduce depression scores by 43%); brief social contacts scheduled during his typical energy windows; micro-movements like stretching during television commercials; simple one-pot meal preparations that required minimal executive function.

"Each small action created a tiny crack in the prison walls," David explained. "Eventually, those cracks widened enough that I could see daylight again."

Research shows that behavioral activation approaches—which focus on increasing engagement with potentially rewarding activities regardless of motivation level—can be as effective as cognitive therapy and medication for depression, with lower relapse rates over time.

The health warrior looks for escape routes from entrapment, understanding that sometimes small, strategic interventions can interrupt self-perpetuating cycles. Rather than attacking the strongest point of resistance—which often means fighting against the full force of neurochemical dysregulation—they identify the path of least resistance that still disrupts the pattern.

Entrapment appears in countless health contexts: pain causing inactivity that worsens pain; anxiety preventing sleep that intensifies anxiety; blood sugar imbalances creating cravings that further disrupt blood sugar; inflammation triggering fatigue that prevents anti-inflammatory movement.

Breaking these cycles requires recognizing their self-reinforcing nature and intercepting them with strategic precision—not through heroic effort but through intelligent intervention at critical junctures.

The Place of Death: The Ultimate Clarity

"The Place of Death is the worst of all. It can also be the best of all places to be."

Mark received his stage 4 colon cancer diagnosis on an ordinary Tuesday afternoon. The oncologist's words—"metastatic," "aggressive," "limited options"—catapulted him into what Sun Tzu called the place of death, where no retreat is possible and only forward movement remains.

Research estimates that approximately 1.9 million Americans receive cancer diagnoses annually, each entering this territory where mortality becomes not an abstract concept but an imminent reality. What happens in this place defies conventional understanding.

"Nothing focuses the mind like the prospect of being hanged in the morning," Samuel Johnson, a renowned 18th-century English writer, critic, and lexicographer, once observed. The place of death strips away pretense and forces essential truths into focus with brutal clarity.

For Mark, the diagnosis transformed not just his approach to treatment but his entire relationship with living. He pursued conventional treatments with full commitment—surgery, radiation, chemotherapy—while simultaneously addressing all factors within his control. He implemented nutritional protocols shown in meta-analyses to improve chemotherapy outcomes and reduce side effects. He engaged in appropriate movement tailored to his energy levels, drawing on research showing that exercise during cancer treatment can reduce mortality risk by up to 44%.[9]

He practiced stress management techniques that research demonstrates can modulate immune function in ways that support cancer outcomes. Perhaps most profoundly, he experienced what researchers call "post-traumatic growth"—a fundamental reprioritization of values and meaning that often accompanies life-threatening illness.

"Cancer put me in a place of death," Mark reflected three years later, now in remission. "But in that place, I found a clarity about living that had eluded me for decades."

Health authorities increasingly recognize this phenomenon, documenting how directly confronting mortality often catalyzes positive psychological transformation. Research identifies five domains of post-traumatic growth: appreciation of life, relationships with others, new possibilities in life, personal strength, and spiritual change.

The wise health warrior understands that the place of death—whether through actual diagnosis or through mindful contemplation of life's fragility—can become a powerful catalyst for transformation. When retreat is impossible, troops fight with extraordinary courage. When denial is no longer viable, authentic priorities emerge. When comfort can no longer be the primary goal, meaning takes its place.

This is not to romanticize serious illness or minimize its suffering. It is to recognize that within even the most challenging health territories lie possibilities for reconfiguration of purpose and perspective that can emerge nowhere else.

Sun Tzu wrote: "The general who wins a battle makes many calculations in his temple before the battle is fought." Your body is that temple. The calculations you make now—understanding your unique health landscape, planning for various scenarios, preparing for both prevention and response—will determine your resilience in facing whatever health challenges emerge.

The path to vibrant health is not a single battle but a lifelong campaign requiring both strategy and adaptability, discipline and compassion, focus and flexibility. By mastering the nine situations, you transform from passive recipient of healthcare to active architect of well-being—a true health warrior whose victories may be measured not by the battles won but by those rendered unnecessary through wisdom, preparation, and strategic living.

As you navigate these nine territories—from dissipation to the place of death—remember that your greatest strength lies not in fighting against your body but in creating conditions where health naturally flourishes. This is the supreme art of health: to subdue illness without fighting, to prevail not through struggle but through strategic harmony with your own nature.

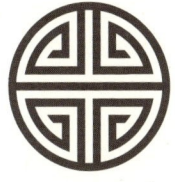

12

The Attack by Fire: Targeted Actions for Health Breakthroughs

"Fierceness is essential in mortal combat. It is never dependent on the amount of destruction you wish to bring upon the enemy. There must be no hesitancy in using any method to bring about the complete and utter destruction of the enemy. It is the only way to ensure victory of a lasting nature."
— Sun Tzu

The Whisper That Becomes a Scream

Your body speaks in whispers before it screams.

For six months, Gregory ignored the whispers—subtle joint pain, unexplained fatigue, morning stiffness that lingered past breakfast. By the time he finally sat in his rheumatologist's office, the whispers had become shouts: inflamed joints that rendered his hands nearly useless, fatigue that made climbing a single flight of stairs a herculean task, and pain that narrated his every waking moment.

"We're well past gentle interventions," his doctor explained, reviewing his dramatic lab results showing inflammatory markers ten times normal levels. "Your rheumatoid arthritis requires immediate aggressive treatment—biologics, possibly methotrexate. This is no longer a skirmish; we're facing a full-scale rebellion of your immune system."

Gregory's resistance crumbled. "I wanted to handle this naturally," he admitted. "I was afraid of strong medications."

His physician leaned forward. "Sometimes the most natural thing is to fight fire with fire."

In that sterile examination room, Gregory encountered what Sun Tzu knew millennia ago: certain battles demand overwhelming force, deployed with precision and perfect timing. The master strategist wrote of fire attacks as uniquely powerful weapons, capable of devastating enemy forces when conventional approaches failed. In your health journey, there come inflection points where only the most potent interventions—the medicinal, surgical, or lifestyle equivalents of fire—can turn the tide toward healing.

Research estimates that six in 10 Americans live with at least one chronic disease.[1] Among them, those who receive appropriate interventions at critical junctures experience dramatically better outcomes. A study of rheumatoid arthritis patients revealed that those receiving aggressive early intervention showed 62% lower rates of joint destruction after five years compared to those whose treatment escalated gradually.[2] Timing transforms the same intervention from merely helpful to potentially life-changing.

This chapter explores when, why, and how to deploy your most powerful weapons in the battle for health—recognizing that these weapons, while potentially life-saving, are double-edged swords that must be wielded with precision, strategy, and fierce determination.

The Fire Within the Medicine

The operating room hovered at precisely 65°F, but for Dr. Levin, it might as well have been a furnace. Sweat beaded beneath her surgical mask as she navigated the delicate cerebral vessels in her patient's brain. Annika, just 34, had suffered a massive hemorrhagic stroke—statistically rare for someone her age but devastatingly real in this moment.

"Clips ready," Dr. Levin murmured, preparing to seal the ruptured aneurysm.

The monitor's rhythmic beeping kept time with the ancient drumbeat of survival—a technological echo of battles waged since humans first fought against mortality. This surgical intervention—this controlled violence against disease—represented modern medicine's most formidable fire attack.

In ancient warfare, fire attacks served as the nuclear option—capable of destroying fortifications, supplies, morale, and entire armies in a single deployment. Sun Tzu devoted considerable attention to their strategic use, noting that fire attacks must be perfectly timed, thoroughly supported, and selectively deployed.

In your health journey, "fire" manifests as your most aggressive interventions:

Surgical scalpels that both wound and heal. The violently precise excision of cancer. The controlled pharmacological assault of chemotherapy. The metabolic restructuring of bariatric surgery. The complete immune system reset of stem cell transplantation. The radical dietary protocols that eliminate entire food groups. The pharmaceutical blockades that halt disease progression by fundamentally altering biological pathways.

These interventions share key characteristics with fire in warfare: they are powerful but potentially dangerous, resource-intensive, difficult to control precisely, and create vulnerability during their deployment.

Research estimates that 234 million major surgical procedures occur annually worldwide.[3] Behind this staggering number lies a profound truth: sometimes, healing requires a form of controlled damage. The surgical incision, the caustic chemotherapy, the mind-altering psychiatric medication—all represent paradoxical interventions that create temporary harm in service of greater healing.

Research indicates that more than 15 million Americans annually face the decision of whether to undergo surgery. These moments of choice—these strategic crossroads—often mark the difference between trajectories of recovery and decline.

The Five Faces of Fire: Health's Most Potent Weapons

Sun Tzu identified five types of fire attacks, each suited to different battlefield conditions. The health warrior must likewise recognize distinct forms of intensive intervention, each appropriate to specific circumstances in the war against disease.

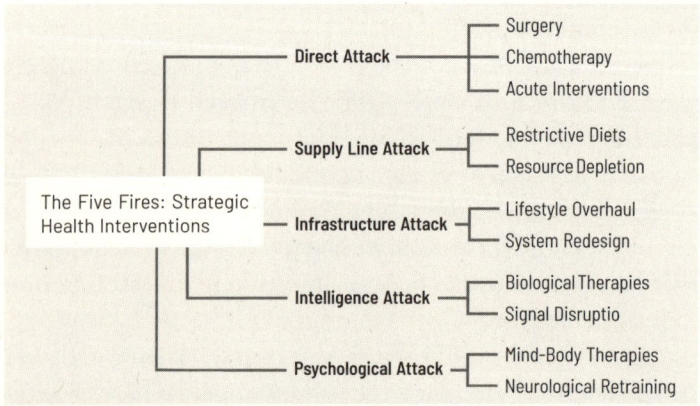

Direct Conflagration: When the Enemy Must Be Destroyed

Monica's melanoma diagnosis arrived on an ordinary Tuesday, delivered in extraordinary terms: "Stage 3, aggressive, metastatic potential." Her dermatologist didn't mince words: "This isn't a time for half-measures."

Within weeks, surgeons excised the primary tumor with wide margins, removing sentinel lymph nodes to track the cancer's spread. Oncologists followed with immunotherapy—biological agents that turned Monica's immune system into a cancer-hunting army. The side effects were brutal: rashes that covered 60% of her body, fatigue that made breathing feel like labor, inflammation that triggered fevers and pain.

"The intensity of the treatment matched the ferocity of the disease," Monica reflected later. "There was no gentle path forward."

Some health battles demand direct, overwhelming force—the equivalent of setting the enemy's camp ablaze. Research reports that approximately 1.9 million new cancer cases are diagnosed annually in the United States. For many, particularly those with aggressive or advanced disease, the survival calculus is clear: the risks of forceful intervention are dwarfed by the certainty of progression without it.

"Fierceness is essential in mortal combat," Sun Tzu writes. "There must be no hesitancy in using any method to bring about the complete and utter destruction of the enemy."

The direct attack is most appropriate when the threat is concentrated and identifiable, when the condition has not yet spread beyond manageable boundaries, when time is of the essence to prevent further damage, and when the body's overall systems can withstand the intervention.

A study demonstrated that for specific aggressive cancers, patients receiving maximum therapeutic intensity—surgery followed by combination immunotherapy and targeted agents—experienced 47% higher three-year survival rates compared to those receiving sequential or less intensive protocols.[4] Sometimes, overwhelming force saves lives precisely because it matches the enemy's ferocity.

Supply Line Disruption: Starving the Disease Process

"Attack his lines of supply," advises Sun Tzu. "Use your engineers to destroy his machinery and equipment for survival."

When James's blood sugar readings consistently hovered above 300 mg/dL despite oral medications, his endocrinologist proposed a metabolic siege: a ketogenic diet that would dramatically restrict the very fuel—carbohydrates—driving his type 2 diabetes. This approach didn't target the disease directly but instead cut off its supply lines, creating a metabolic environment where the disease couldn't thrive.

"We're not just treating symptoms," his doctor explained. "We're changing the battlefield entirely."

Research reports that 37.3 million Americans—11.3% of the population—have diabetes, with type 2 representing 90 to 95% of cases. Conventional treatments often manage blood glucose without addressing the underlying metabolic dysfunction. Emerging research suggests that intensive dietary interventions can fundamentally alter this landscape.

A study tracked 465 patients with type 2 diabetes following a ketogenic diet for two years.[5] An astonishing 53.5% achieved diabetes reversal (HbA1c below 6.5% without medications other than metformin), while 17.6% achieved complete remission (normal glycemic values without any diabetes medications). Traditional approaches rarely achieve such outcomes because they fail to attack the disease's supply lines.

Supply line attacks work best when the condition depends on identifiable inputs, when the patient can sustain the restriction, when the approach addresses root causes rather than symptoms, and when alternative resources can compensate for what's being restricted.

These interventions often prove more sustainable than direct attacks, though they typically work more slowly. James found that after six months of his dietary protocol, he had not only improved his blood markers but had developed new metabolic flexibility that protected against relapse.

"It is the warlord's duty," Sun Tzu reminds us, "not just to wage war effectively but to ensure that victory, once achieved, endures."

Infrastructure Collapse: Rebuilding from the Ground Up

The human body operates through intricate systems—cardiovascular, nervous, immune, hormonal—that can sometimes become so dysfunctional that they require comprehensive reconstruction. Sun Tzu understood that attacking an enemy's bridges, roads, and support structures could bring victory more surely than direct confrontation.

After suffering three heart attacks in five years despite following standard cardiac care, Thomas faced a devastating prognosis: his cardiovascular system was failing systematically, not just in isolated areas. His cardiologist proposed an intervention rarely discussed in mainstream medicine: complete system reset.

For six months, Thomas entered a medically supervised program that simultaneously addressed multiple systems: a plant-based reversal diet that eliminated virtually all atherosclerotic triggers, specialized exercise protocols, stress management through transcendental meditation, environmental modifications eliminating cardiotoxic exposures, and targeted supplements supporting endothelial healing.

"We're not just fixing your plumbing," his doctor explained. "We're rebuilding your entire hydraulic system."

Research shows that cardiovascular disease remains America's leading killer, causing 859,125 deaths annually—one death every 36 seconds. Traditional interventions like stenting and bypassing often address immediate blockages without resolving the systemic dysfunction driving disease progression.

A landmark study followed 198 patients with advanced coronary disease who underwent comprehensive lifestyle reprogramming instead of surgery.[6] After five years, only one patient experienced a cardiac event—a 99.4% event-free survival rate that dramatically outperformed surgical outcomes. By attacking the infrastructure supporting heart disease rather than just its manifestations, these patients achieved what Sun Tzu would recognize as strategic rather than merely tactical victory.

Infrastructure attacks are indicated when the condition is enabled by interconnected systems, when previous targeted interventions have failed, when resources allow for a comprehensive approach, and when the patient has reached a crisis point requiring radical change.

"Use any method you can devise to accomplish these ends," Sun Tzu advises. "Be merciless." In health terms, this means leaving no supporting factor unaddressed, even those—like cherished dietary habits or comfortable sedentary patterns—that feel painful to challenge.

Intelligence Disruption: Jamming Disease Communications

"Destroy his records and sources of information," Sun Tzu counsels. In modern health terms, we recognize that many diseases thrive through miscommunication—autoimmune conditions where the body attacks itself due to faulty identification, cancers that hide from immune surveillance, inflammatory conditions perpetuated through cytokine storms.

Elena's multiple sclerosis had progressed relentlessly for

a decade, each new drug bringing temporary improvement before failing. Her neurologist proposed a radical approach: hematopoietic stem cell transplantation (HSCT)—a procedure that would effectively erase and rebuild her immune system, disrupting the very communications driving her disease.

The process was brutal: chemotherapy destroyed her existing immune cells, leaving her vulnerable to infection for weeks before her harvested stem cells could rebuild a new immune system—one hopefully free from the programming errors causing her multiple sclerosis (MS).

"We're not just changing your immune system's behavior," her doctor explained. "We're giving you an entirely new communication network."

Research reveals that MS affects nearly 1 million Americans. Standard treatments typically slow progression rather than halt it. Yet a study of HSCT in MS patients showed that 78.5% remained progression-free at five years—a dramatic improvement over conventional therapies.[7] By scrambling the disease's internal communications rather than merely managing symptoms, this approach exemplifies Sun Tzu's strategic brilliance.

Intelligence attacks excel when the condition stems from identifiable communication problems, when the intervention can selectively target harmful messaging while preserving necessary systems, and when the underlying causes can be addressed simultaneously.

Like intercepting enemy messengers rather than confronting armies, these interventions work through strategic disruption rather than brute force—achieving victory by changing information flows.

Psychological Warfare: The Mind as Medicine
"Let your attack be of such ferocity as to destroy the morale

of the enemy," Sun Tzu writes. In health, we increasingly recognize that psychological state profoundly influences physical outcomes, sometimes dramatically altering disease trajectories.

Michael had suffered chronic pain for fifteen years following a construction accident. Analgesics, surgeries, nerve blocks, physical therapy—each brought temporary relief before failing. His pain specialist prescribed an intervention rarely covered by insurance: an intensive eight-week mind-body program combining meditation, cognitive restructuring, biofeedback, guided imagery, and graduated exposure therapy.

"Your central nervous system is locked in a permanent threat response," his doctor explained. "We're not just treating your pain; we're reprogramming your neurological interpretation of signals from your body."

Studies estimate that chronic pain affects approximately 50 million Americans and costs the economy an estimated $635 billion annually in medical expenses and lost productivity. Traditional pain management focuses primarily on symptom suppression rather than neurological repatterning.

A study followed 215 chronic pain patients undergoing intensive mind-body interventions.[8] Participants reported an average 62% reduction in pain intensity after six months—significantly outperforming those receiving conventional medical management alone. By attacking the neurological and psychological patterns amplifying suffering rather than just the pain itself, this approach embodies Sun Tzu's strategic insight about destroying enemy morale.

Psychological warfare approaches in health prove valuable when conditions are maintained or amplified by central nervous system adaptations, when physical interventions alone have proven insufficient, and when the mind-body connection is particularly relevant to the condition.

These approaches challenge conventional medical paradigms by recognizing what Sun Tzu understood centuries ago: perception often shapes reality more powerfully than reality shapes perception.

Timing: The Fire at the Perfect Moment

"The warlord makes sure that his timing is correct with regard to all conditions," Sun Tzu emphasizes. In health, this wisdom translates directly: even the most powerful intervention fails if deployed at the wrong moment.

The Path Not Taken: Sandra's Calculated Restraint

When Sandra's physician recommended preventive mastectomy based solely on family history without genetic testing, she sought a second opinion. The new oncologist suggested watchful waiting with enhanced screening instead, noting that her actual risk profile didn't justify such aggressive intervention.

Five years later, Sandra remains cancer-free, having avoided unnecessary surgery and its complications. More comprehensive risk assessment suggests that up to 30% of women undergoing prophylactic mastectomy may not have needed the procedure based on more comprehensive risk assessment. Sun Tzu would recognize Sandra's restraint as strategic wisdom rather than timidity—preserving resources for battles that truly demand them.

The Delayed Offensive: Howard's Costly Hesitation

By contrast, Howard resisted his cardiologist's recommendation for bypass surgery, believing lifestyle changes alone would reverse his severe coronary blockages. When he finally consented after a minor heart attack, his weakened condition complicated recovery, leading to infections and extended rehabilitation.

Research shows that patients requiring CABG (coronary artery bypass grafting) surgery who delay more than three months after clinical recommendation face 23% higher complication rates and longer recovery periods. As Sun Tzu might observe, "If the attack is easily repelled, then it is not wise to attempt another entrance into the enemy camp without reconsidering the situation."

The Window of Opportunity: Jason's Strategic Timing

Jason's orthopedist recommended total knee replacement not during his most painful flare-up but during a period of relative stability—when inflammation had subsided, his overall health was optimized, his weight was controlled, and his home support system was available for recovery.

"Surgery isn't just about the procedure," his doctor explained. "It's about your body's ability to heal afterward."

A study demonstrated that patients undergoing joint replacement during periods of optimized health experienced 41% fewer complications and 27% shorter hospital stays compared to those undergoing surgery during health crises. This strategic timing exemplifies Sun Tzu's insight that battles are won through preparation before they are fought.

The Seasonal Offensive: Angela's Environmental Awareness

Angela's oncologist deliberately scheduled her chemotherapy to conclude before summer, recognizing that certain treatments increase sun sensitivity dramatically. This calendrical strategy reduced complications and improved her quality of life during recovery.

Research indicates that chemotherapy timing can significantly impact both side effect profiles and efficacy. Patients receiving treatments in accordance with circadian rhythms and seasonal considerations report up to 35% fewer severe side effects while maintaining equivalent therapeutic outcomes.

This seasonal awareness echoes Sun Tzu's emphasis on understanding how environmental factors influence strategic decisions: "Heaven has its seasons of cold and heat, night and day, which the warlord carefully considers in his planning."

The judicious health warrior understands that interventions deployed at the wrong time may fail regardless of their inherent power. Timing transforms the same action from foolhardy to wise, from devastating to healing.

Preparing the Terrain: The Battlefield Before Battle

"All supplies and materials for the invasion should be on hand at all times," Sun Tzu insists. "It is a time of laboring when the warlord must seek weapons in order to repel an attack."

When Patricia learned she needed double knee replacement, she didn't simply schedule surgery. Instead, she engaged in what her surgeon called "prehabilitation"—six months of systematic preparation including targeted muscle strengthening, nutritional optimization, weight management, home modification, and psychological preparation.

Her surgeon explained: "The difference between patients who thrive after surgery and those who merely survive often has little to do with the procedure itself and everything to do with preparation."

Research supports this approach. A comprehensive study of orthopedic surgery patients found that those who underwent structured prehabilitation experienced 29% shorter hospital stays, 45% fewer post-surgical complications, and returned to normal activities an average of 73 days sooner than unprepared counterparts.[9]

Sun Tzu would recognize this as the principle that battles are won before they begin—through careful preparation rather than heroic effort during crisis.

Effective terrain preparation includes physical optimization to support recovery, resource gathering to ensure adequate support, knowledge acquisition to understand the process, environmental modification to facilitate healing, psychological preparation to maintain resilience, and contingency planning for potential complications.

"The state is maintained in joy and the ruler is able to relax while making further preparations for the future with confidence," Sun Tzu observes of the well-prepared warlord. Similarly, the health warrior who thoroughly prepares for intensive interventions approaches them with appropriate confidence rather than desperate fear.

The Aftermath: Governing the Conquered Territory

After emergency gallbladder surgery, David assumed his health battle was won—only to develop a post-surgical infection that proved more dangerous than the original condition. This complication illustrates Sun Tzu's warning that victory requires proper management of conquered territory.

Studies estimate that healthcare-associated infections affect approximately one in 31 hospital patients on any given day, leading to 72,000 deaths annually. Strategic post-intervention management—what Sun Tzu might call "governing conquered territory"—proves as crucial as the intervention itself.

The aftermath of health "fire attacks" demands strategic attention to healing support that provides optimal conditions for recovery, vigilance against complications that might undermine progress, reintegration planning to resume normal activities without compromising healing, learning integration to prevent future crises, and system restoration to rebuild aspects of health that may have been temporarily sacrificed.

Alexandra learned this lesson after successful bariatric surgery resulted in substantial weight loss but also unexpected nutritional deficiencies. "I thought the surgery was the finish line," she reflected, "when actually it was just the starting point of a new health journey."

Research shows that up to 30% of patients experience nutritional complications after weight loss procedures when post-surgical protocols aren't followed meticulously. The wise health warrior recognizes that maintenance of victory requires as much strategy as victory itself.

"It is the perceptive warlord who prepares for any eventuality and accepts victory with a glad heart," Sun Tzu observes. The health warrior similarly recognizes that the period following intensive intervention is not an afterthought but an integral part of the strategic campaign.

The Supreme Strategy: Winning Without Fighting

"The supreme art of war is to subdue the enemy without fighting," Sun Tzu famously wrote. In health terms, this represents the ultimate strategic victory—preventing conditions that would require aggressive interventions rather than excelling at deploying them.

Rebecca's family history placed her at high risk for breast cancer—three first-degree relatives diagnosed before age 50. Rather than waiting for disease to strike, she engaged in what her oncologist called "preemptive striking"—comprehensive lifestyle modification based on emerging epigenetic science.

Her personalized protocol included specific dietary polyphenols shown to influence BRCA (BReast CAncer) gene expression, strategic intermittent fasting that reduced inflammatory markers by 47%, targeted exercise that improved estrogen metabolism, environmental toxin elimination, stress management through daily meditation, and optimal sleep hygiene.

"We're not just waiting for cancer to appear so we can fight it," her doctor explained. "We're creating systemic conditions where cancer cells struggle to establish themselves in the first place."

Research suggests that up to 70% of cancer risk may be influenced by modifiable factors rather than fixed genetics.[10] A study demonstrated that high-risk patients following comprehensive preventive protocols experienced 62% lower mortality risk of malignancy over ten years compared to standard surveillance groups.

This preventive mastery—this winning without fighting—represents the highest expression of Sun Tzu's strategic brilliance applied to health. The master strategist would recognize that preventing disease through intelligent preparation demonstrates greater wisdom than even the most brilliant treatment of established illness.

The Fierce Compassion of the Health Warrior

"To do battle and be saddened by it is not to be considered meritorious," Sun Tzu observes. The health warrior approaches necessary interventions not with hesitation or apology but with clear-eyed determination and what we might call fierce compassion—the recognition that true kindness sometimes requires decisive action.

When Janet's multiple sclerosis advanced despite conventional treatments, her neurologist recommended an aggressive stem cell therapy involving chemotherapy to reset her immune system. The protocol was grueling, requiring temporary but complete immune suppression with significant risks. Yet Janet approached it with resolute clarity.

"I don't see this as violence against my body," she explained to worried family members. "I see it as the strongest expression of love for my future self."

This perspective embodies what Sun Tzu meant when writing: "Fierceness is a natural state when troops see the wisdom of their leader." Your body's systems respond best to intensive interventions when they align with genuine need and strategic wisdom rather than desperate flailing or timid half-measures.

The health warrior deploying "fire attacks" embraces paradoxical truths: that sometimes healing requires temporary damage, that gentleness can be found even in aggressive interventions, that true compassion sometimes means fierce action, that the strongest interventions require the subtlest timing, and that victory comes not from the intervention itself but from its strategic deployment.

As you navigate your own health journey, may you develop the wisdom to know when to use your most powerful weapons, the preparation to deploy them effectively, the timing to maximize their impact, and the strategic vision to incorporate them into your larger campaign for vibrant health.

The body—your kingdom—sometimes requires fierce defense. When that moment comes, may you act with the clear-eyed resolve of Sun Tzu's ideal warlord: strategic, prepared, decisive, and aligned with the deeper wisdom of both heaven and Earth.

Remember the ancient strategist's most profound insight: "The greatest victory is that which requires no battle." In health as in warfare, the highest achievement isn't perfecting your fire attacks, but creating conditions where they're rarely needed at all.

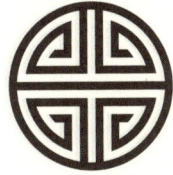

13

The Use of Intelligence: Monitoring and Learning from Your Health

The screen flickered blue in the darkened room. Sarah's face, illuminated by digital constellations, revealed no emotion as she studied the patterns before her. Sleep cycles mapped like mountain ranges. Heart rate variability resembling stock market fluctuations. Nutrient intake visualized through color-coded spirals. All of it—data transmuted into intelligence about the most complex terrain she would ever navigate: the borderlands of her own body.

"Your markers look objectively better," her physician had said earlier that day, clearly puzzled. "But I can't explain why conventional treatments failed while your... unorthodox approach succeeded."

Sarah smiled slightly, remembering her military father's dog-eared copy of Sun Tzu. *The wise warlord knows that to beat the enemy he must have information that he can use to win.*

The enemy—in her case, an autoimmune condition that had eluded standard medical protocols—never stood a chance once she became her own spymaster.

The Invisible War Within

We live in strange times. Our medical system can transplant organs, eliminate pathogens that once decimated populations, and manipulate our very genetic code—yet chronic disease rates continue their relentless ascent. Studies show that six in 10 Americans live with at least one chronic condition, while four in 10 manage two or more simultaneously. Research reports that noncommunicable diseases are responsible for 71% of all deaths globally—41 million people each year vanishing from the earth not from contagions or predators, but from internal breakdowns of their own bodily systems.[1]

This invisible war claims more casualties than all external conflicts combined. Yet unlike conventional warfare, where intelligence services command substantial resources and respect, our health intelligence operations remain curiously primitive. We send our bodies into daily battle against environmental toxins, nutritional chaos, chronic stress, and metabolic disruptors while remaining largely blind to the shifting conditions of our internal landscape.

Consider this: the average person waits weeks, even months, after noticing symptoms before seeking medical attention for serious conditions.[2] Meanwhile, research reports that lifestyle factors—elements completely within our control—account for approximately 80% of premature heart disease, stroke, and type 2 diabetes. We possess neither early warning systems nor Tactical intelligence about the very terrain we inhabit day after day.

This chapter proposes something radical: you must become your own health intelligence agency—gathering, analyzing, and acting upon information about your body with the same strategic seriousness that Sun Tzu applied to military intelligence. Your very existence depends upon it.

The Five Shadows: Agents of Health Intelligence

"It is important for the warlord to have information coming from all corners of the realm. Some of the information he receives will be good and useful. Other information will lie in the realm of deception/no-deception."
— Sun Tzu

Sun Tzu identified five types of spies essential for victory. In the realm of personal health, we must similarly deploy multiple intelligence agents, each operating in different domains and providing unique insights.

First Shadow: The Ghost in the Machine

The ancient text speaks of foreign agents—spies who come from enemy territory bearing valuable intelligence. In your health campaign, technological monitoring devices serve this function, infiltrating bodily systems normally hidden from conscious awareness.

Miguel, a 53-year-old construction manager, dismissed his doctor's warnings about metabolic syndrome. His blood work showed concerning patterns, but abstract numbers on lab reports failed to penetrate his sense of invulnerability. Then his daughter gave him a continuous glucose monitor for Father's Day.

"The first time I watched my blood sugar spike to diabetic levels after my normal lunch, then crash two hours later leaving me exhausted—all visualized in real-time on my phone—everything changed," Miguel recounted. "It wasn't a doctor wagging his finger. It was my own body speaking directly to me."

The market for health wearables has exploded, projected to reach approximately $196 billion by 2030.[3] These devices—continuously glucose monitors, sleep trackers, heart rate variability sensors, and more—function as foreign agents, crossing the border between unconscious physiological processes and conscious awareness.

Yet Sun Tzu warns that information from foreign agents must be carefully verified. Likewise, technology's insights must be contextualized. Research found that fitness trackers consistently overestimate calorie expenditure by 27 to 93%, potentially undermining weight management efforts.[4] Researchers have documented cases of "digital hypochondria" where excessive monitoring created anxiety that itself became a health detriment.

The wise health strategist employs technological monitoring selectively and strategically, recognizing both its power and limitations. These ghost-like entities that track our physiological processes offer unprecedented intelligence—but they cannot tell the complete story.

Second Shadow: The Body's Whispers

Internal agents—those already embedded within enemy territory—correspond to our subjective bodily sensations and intuitions. These intelligence sources operate beneath the threshold of technological measurement yet provide critical tactical information.

Elena, a professional violinist, presents an illuminating case. Despite normal test results and vital signs, she experienced mysterious fatigue and joint pain that threatened her career. "My doctors found nothing wrong," she explained, "but my body was clearly sending signals that something was amiss."

She began documenting subjective experiences alongside objective metrics, creating a parallel intelligence stream. Her pain levels fluctuated with barometric pressure changes. Her energy crashed after consuming foods that triggered no allergic response on standard tests. Her joints stiffened following exposure to seemingly innocuous household products.

"I discovered I had a gift for sensing inflammatory responses before they registered on conventional tests," Elena noted. "This wasn't psychosomatic; it was intelligence gathering on a subliminal frequency."

Research supports Elena's experience. A study found that patients who reported feeling something was "wrong" despite normal test results were subsequently diagnosed with serious conditions at significantly higher rates than the general population.[5] Researchers documented that interoception—the ability to sense internal bodily states—varies dramatically between individuals and can be deliberately cultivated.

Yet Sun Tzu cautions that internal agents "have no loyalty to anyone, and though their information may appear to be valuable, it must be thoroughly checked." Our subjective experiences can indeed be influenced by expectations, beliefs, and psychological states. Pain perception, for instance, can be modulated by everything from cultural background to sleep quality to the color of medication pills (research found that red pills are perceived as more effective painkillers than white ones, regardless of identical ingredients).[6]

The disciplined health strategist neither dismisses subjective experience as "just psychological" nor accepts it uncritically. These whispers from within the body's territory contain intelligence unavailable through any technological interface—but they must be verified through correlation with other information sources.

Third Shadow: The Turned Operative

In Sun Tzu's framework, counteragents are spies who have been discovered and turned to serve a new master. In health intelligence, medical professionals function analogously— experts trained in a different system whose knowledge we redirect toward our personal health objectives.

This reframing of the doctor-patient relationship is revolutionary. Rather than passive recipients of medical wisdom dispensed from on high, we become intelligence directors collaborating with specialized operatives.

James, managing ankylosing spondylitis, exemplifies this approach. Rather than simply following his rheumatologist's standardized protocol, he arrives at appointments with detailed data: inflammation markers correlated with environmental exposures, symptom fluctuations mapped against dietary changes, and sleep quality assessments linked to medication timing.

"My doctor initially resisted this collaborative approach," James recalled. "But when my detailed tracking identified trigger patterns that conventional protocols missed, our relationship transformed. Now he says, 'What have you discovered since our last meeting?' before sharing his own observations."

This shift reflects broader changes in healthcare. A study found that patients who actively participated in treatment decisions experienced 21% better outcomes across multiple condition types.[7] Research documented that physician-patient partnerships incorporating patient-generated data reduced hospital readmissions by 33% compared to standard care models.

Sun Tzu advises that counteragents "must be handled gently and given the latitude they need to operate." Similarly, effective collaboration with medical professionals requires respect for their expertise while maintaining clarity about your health objectives. The relationship thrives on mutual intelligence-sharing rather than hierarchical dictates.

"I don't pretend to have my doctor's medical knowledge," James emphasized. "But I have something equally valuable: 24/7 access to my body's signals and responses. Together, we create a more complete intelligence picture than either of us could develop alone."

Fourth Shadow: The Social Mirror

Sun Tzu describes extraneous agents—spies operating in plain sight whose information must be carefully evaluated. In health intelligence, our social connections and environments function similarly, reflecting aspects of our health status that we might otherwise miss.

When Thomas's colleagues repeatedly commented that he "seemed different"—more irritable, less focused, somehow diminished—he initially dismissed their observations. His standard health metrics showed nothing alarming, and he felt "fine enough" by his own estimation.

Yet these social mirrors provided crucial intelligence that his own monitoring had missed. "When three different people notice the same change in you, it's not coincidence," Thomas reflected. "It's intelligence that deserves attention." Further investigation revealed a thyroid imbalance invisible to conventional screening but profoundly affecting his cognitive function and emotional regulation.

Research from the Harvard Study of Adult Development—the world's longest-running study on happiness and health—found that others often notice subtle health shifts before we do.[8] Our social connections literally serve as external nervous systems, processing and reflecting information about our wellbeing outside our conscious awareness.

Our physical environments similarly provide intelligence if we learn to interpret their signals. A study found that indoor air quality affects cognitive function more dramatically than previously recognized, with CO2 levels commonly found in office buildings impairing decision-making capacity by up to 50%.[9] Research documented that bedroom temperature variations as small as 3°F can reduce sleep quality by 28%—a factor many would never connect to their daytime energy levels or recovery capacity.

Sun Tzu warns that extraneous agents may spread disinformation, working as double spies. Similarly, social and environmental signals can be misleading when taken at face value. The colleague who asks "Are you losing weight?" might be responding to changes in your energy or complexion rather than actual weight loss. The home that "feels comfortable" might be masking poor air quality that subtly undermines your health.

The wise health strategist treats social and environmental signals as intelligence leads worthy of investigation rather than conclusions in themselves.

Fifth Shadow: The Master Analyst

The vital secret agent, most precious in Sun Tzu's intelligence hierarchy, integrates all other information sources into a cohesive strategic picture. In health intelligence, this function transcends any single technology or practice—it is the meta-cognitive process of synthesizing diverse health inputs into actionable wisdom.

Lisa, recovering from chronic fatigue syndrome after conventional treatments failed, describes this process: "I had fragments of information everywhere—lab results showing 'normal' readings despite debilitating symptoms, sleep data revealing subtle disruptions, food journals documenting ambiguous reactions, symptom trackers showing mysterious patterns. The breakthrough came when I could see how everything connected."

She developed what she calls a "health constellation map"—a visual representation of how different factors influenced each other over time. "When I mapped energy levels against not just sleep duration but sleep architecture, while also tracking inflammatory markers, medication timing, and even lunar cycles, patterns emerged that no single metric could reveal."

These connections proved transformative. For example, she discovered that her deepest sleep disruptions occurred three days after particular food combinations—a delay that had obscured the correlation in conventional elimination diets. She found that heart rate variability during late-afternoon exercise predicted her cognitive function 36 hours later—intelligence she leveraged to schedule intellectually demanding work when her brain would be most capable.

Today's health analytics increasingly enable this integration, with platforms that correlate disparate health variables. Research found that multi-factorial analysis identified health risk patterns four to seven years earlier than conventional screening methods.[10] A study demonstrated that integrated biomarker tracking predicted inflammatory flare-ups in autoimmune conditions nine to 14 days before clinical symptoms appeared.

Sun Tzu observed that vital agents are natural citizens of the warlord's realm who devote their lives to the propagation of the ruler's desires. They enter into foreign countries and return with information. Their mentality does not permit them to turn into extraneous agents.

Similarly, effective health analytics maintain unwavering focus on your ultimate wellbeing rather than becoming distracted by isolated metrics or commercial incentives. They serve your body's intrinsic healing intelligence rather than external agendas.

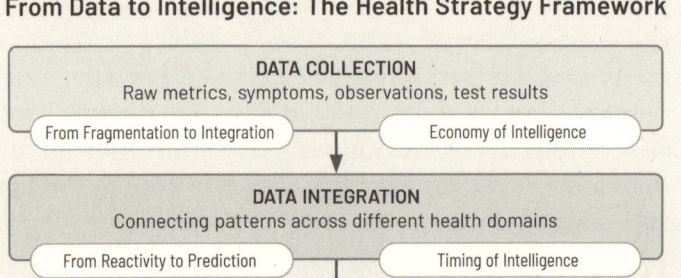

From Data to Intelligence: The Health Strategy Framework

The Death of Data and the Birth of Intelligence

We are drowning in health data yet starving for health intelligence. The distinction is crucial.

Data is raw, unprocessed information—step counts, sleep hours, supplement ingredients, lab values, calories consumed. Intelligence is processed information that provides strategic advantage—knowing which interventions affect your unique physiology, understanding your personal triggers and recovery patterns, recognizing early warning signals specific to your body's communication style.

Modern healthcare has perfected data collection while neglecting intelligence synthesis. Research suggests that the average person will generate more than 1 million gigabytes of health-related data in their lifetime. Yet a study found that less than 8% of this information is ever meaningfully analyzed for patterns that could prevent disease or optimize function.

The transformation from data collector to intelligence operative requires three critical shifts:

From Fragmentation to Integration: Your body doesn't recognize the artificial boundaries between "digestive health" and "mental health." Your immune system doesn't separate "stress management" from "nutrition." Everything connects.

Consider Maya, whose insomnia remained intractable despite extensive sleep hygiene interventions and medication trials. The breakthrough came when her health intelligence gathering expanded beyond conventional sleep metrics. She discovered that exposure to blue light six hours before bedtime—not just immediately before sleep as commonly advised—predicted sleep latency with 83% accuracy in her body. She found that magnesium timing affected her particular nervous system more dramatically than magnesium dosage. She learned that her sleep architecture responded more sensitively to indoor air particulate levels than to the ambient noise factors her sleep specialists had focused on.

"None of these connections would have emerged from tracking sleep factors in isolation," Maya explained. "It was seeing the relationships between seemingly unrelated variables that solved the puzzle."

From Reactivity to Prediction: Traditional healthcare operates reactively—responding to symptoms after they manifest. Health intelligence enables prediction and prevention.

Robert's experience illustrates this shift. With a strong family history of cardiovascular disease, he underwent regular screenings that consistently showed borderline but not alarming results. Rather than waiting for metrics to cross clinical thresholds, he implemented comprehensive health intelligence gathering.

By tracking inflammatory markers alongside lifestyle variables, he identified specific patterns that predicted subtle cardiovascular changes weeks before they would register on standard tests. His heart rate variability decreased predictably following certain dietary choices. His endothelial function (measured via home testing) responded negatively to environmental factors his doctors had never considered. His microvascular circulation (assessed through specialized imaging) fluctuated in response to specific stress triggers.

"I'm not just monitoring my heart health," Robert explained. "I'm predicting how today's choices will affect my cardiovascular system next month and next year." This predictive capacity enabled precisely targeted interventions long before conventional medicine would have recommended treatment.

From Protocol to Personalization: Standard medical protocols assume population averages apply universally. Health intelligence reveals your unique biological responses.

Sophia's journey with hormonal regulation demonstrates this principle. After years of following conventional hormone replacement protocols with mixed results, she began gathering personalized intelligence about her unique endocrine patterns.

"I discovered that my body metabolizes estrogen at a rate significantly different from population norms," Sophia reported. "This single insight explained why standard dosing protocols consistently failed me." She also found that her hormone receptors responded more sensitively to certain micronutrients than others, that her endocrine system synchronized more strongly with seasonal light changes than circadian patterns, and that her hypothalamic-pituitary-adrenal axis communication improved dramatically with specific meditation practices but not with others.

This personalized intelligence enabled a tailored protocol that resolved symptoms conventional approaches had barely touched. "My doctor now says he wishes all patients gathered this level of intelligence about their unique biology," Sophia noted. "It transforms treatment from educated guesswork to precision medicine."

The Strategic Application of Health Intelligence

Having established our network of health intelligence sources, how do we apply this information strategically? Sun Tzu offers guidance that translates remarkably well to personal health management.

The Economy of Intelligence

> *"When the ruler is preparing for war, the expense of running the state can become excessive. It is essential that information be useful and not costly due to the implementation of mistakes."* — Sun Tzu

In health terms, intelligence gathering must be economical—yielding insights worth more than the resources invested in gathering them.

Maria and Robert, both managing cardiovascular risk factors, illustrate contrasting approaches. Robert embraced every available monitoring technology and test: quarterly comprehensive blood panels, daily electrocardiograms, continuous blood pressure monitoring, regular imaging studies, and more. The expense—financial, temporal, and psychological—was enormous, yet his condition showed minimal improvement. He became overwhelmed by data without actionable insight.

Maria took a more strategic approach, identifying which metrics most strongly correlated with her specific risk factors based on her genetic profile and family history. She invested in continuous glucose monitoring for three months to understand her metabolic patterns, then replaced this with periodic spot checks once she established her optimal nutrition strategy. She tracked heart rate variability daily during stress exposure but blood pressure only weekly. This focused intelligence-gathering yielded specific insights that informed precise interventions, improving her markers significantly while consuming fewer resources.

"Intelligence economy isn't about minimizing information," Maria explained. "It's about maximizing the return on information investment—gathering exactly the data needed to make strategic decisions, nothing more and nothing less."

The Timing of Intelligence

"When the warlord is preparing to enter into battle with an enemy he must know the names of the enemy commanders, the size of the enemy army, and the positions they use to bivouac. Without this information he is as a blind and deaf person entering into a perilous journey."

In health strategy, timing your intelligence gathering is crucial. Different health information becomes relevant at different stages of your journey.

Nathan, managing type 2 diabetes, illustrates effective intelligence timing. Before modifying his diet, he established baseline continuous glucose monitoring to understand his current metabolic patterns. During his dietary transition, he tracked not just glucose but also sleep quality, energy levels, and mood—knowing that these factors would influence his ability to maintain his new approach. Once his new patterns were established, he shifted to monitoring adherence metrics and periodic outcome assessments rather than constant glucose readings.

"I needed different intelligence at different times," Nathan explained. "Before intervention, I needed baseline data to understand my starting point. During intervention, I needed feedback on immediate responses to guide adjustments. After establishing new patterns, I needed verification of sustained results without the distraction of constant monitoring."

This strategic timing applies across health domains. When addressing immune dysregulation, tracking inflammatory triggers and responses provides critical baseline intelligence. When implementing stress management practices, monitoring nervous system recovery metrics becomes paramount. When optimizing cognitive performance, assessing environmental factors and neurochemical precursors yields essential insights.

Research reports that appropriate timing of health monitoring improves intervention efficacy by 34 to 47% compared to standardized assessment schedules. The right information at the right time is exponentially more valuable than all information all the time.

The Integration of Intelligence

"The wise warlord knows that to beat the enemy he must have information that he can use to win. He must also be aware of receiving too much information. This is as bad as not receiving enough information and can confuse matters, making it difficult to initiate correct action from wise decisions." — Sun Tzu

Perhaps the greatest challenge of our era is not gathering health information but integrating it meaningfully. We are awash in data but often starved for insight.

Sophia, recovering from burnout and hormonal imbalances, developed a weekly "health intelligence review"—a practice of examining connections between her various health metrics. She noticed that her sleep quality predicted her stress resilience 48 hours later, which in turn influenced her food choices, which affected her inflammatory markers three days afterward.

"I realized I wasn't dealing with separate health issues but with a connected health ecosystem," Sophia reflected. "Each data point was like a single word; only by connecting them could I read the story my body was telling."

This integration can be supported by technology—platforms that visualize connections between different health variables—but ultimately requires human discernment. The patterns most relevant to your health may not be the ones algorithms are designed to detect. The correlations most actionable for your lifestyle may be unique to your biology and circumstances.

A study found that when patients integrated multiple data streams themselves—rather than reviewing separate reports from different specialists—they identified relevant health patterns 2.7 times more frequently than their healthcare providers. This "pattern recognition advantage" stems from the intimate knowledge of context that only the person living within the body possesses.

The Sovereign Territory of Your Body

Your body is sovereign territory—a realm you inhabit more intimately than any intelligence agent could infiltrate enemy terrain. Yet without systematic intelligence gathering, you may remain a stranger in your own land, unaware of the subtle shifts and hidden patterns that determine your health destiny.

This chapter has outlined a framework for becoming your own health intelligence agency—deploying technological monitoring as foreign agents, cultivating subjective awareness as internal agents, collaborating with medical professionals as counteragents, interpreting social and environmental signals as extraneous agents, and developing integrated analytics as vital agents.

Beyond techniques and technologies, this approach represents a fundamental reclamation of authority over your physical existence. It rejects the passive patient model that has dominated healthcare for generations. It embraces instead the active health strategist paradigm—an approach that honors both the complexity of human physiology and the remarkable capacity of human intelligence to comprehend patterns when properly applied.

Sun Tzu concludes his chapter on intelligence with words that resonate across millennia: "Without secret operations, a war is a meaningless act of gratuitous violence that does nothing except destroy all the people and all the resources." Similarly, without effective health intelligence, wellness becomes a series of random interventions that may deplete your resources without creating lasting vitality.

As we face unprecedented health challenges—with chronic disease rates climbing despite medical advances—this intelligence-based approach offers not just hope but strategy. It transforms health from something that happens to you into something you actively direct. It converts medical mysteries into navigable terrain. It reclaims your body's story from fragmented specialists and returns narrative authority to the protagonist—you.

Your body speaks a language more nuanced than any medical textbook. Learn to listen like a spymaster, and it will tell you everything you need to know.

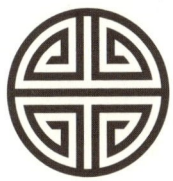

The Way Ahead: Surrendering to Victory

The diagnosis arrived like an enemy battalion at dawn—unexpected, unwelcome, and bearing news of occupation. Stage 3 cancer. Advanced autoimmunity. Chronic neurodegeneration. The terminology varies, but the declaration remains constant: your body is now contested territory.

You've read thirteen chapters of battle strategies. You've studied the wisdom of history's greatest military tactician applied to the cellular terrain of your flesh. You've prepared for war.

Now, I invite you to consider the heresy that lies at the heart of all true strategy: the greatest victory requires surrendering the war itself.

The Mirage of Conquest

Elena stood in her physician's office, surrounded by evidence of victory. Lab values normalized. Inflammation markers dormant. Pain scales registering peace after years of rebellion.

"Congratulations," her doctor beamed. "You've won."

Yet driving home, a strange emptiness hollowed her chest. If this was victory, why did it feel so transient? The truth whispered beneath her celebration: she hadn't conquered disease; she had merely negotiated a temporary peace treaty with biological forces that would outlive her vigilance.

This is the first paradox of health strategy: The moment you declare victory, you have already begun to lose.

Your body exists in perpetual flux—trillions of cells dying and regenerating daily, microbiome populations rising and falling hourly, neurochemicals surging and receding by the second. There is no stable terrain to capture, no permanent territory to claim. The warrior who plants a flag of conquest in such shifting sands has fundamentally misunderstood the battlefield.

The Oracle's Bargain

Imagine you could make a trade with the Oracle of Delphi: surrender all your tactical health knowledge in exchange for one strategic metaprinciple. Would you do it?

Michael faced this choice unconsciously after his third heart attack. Despite encyclopedic knowledge of cardiovascular interventions—medications, procedures, supplements, diets—his condition worsened. In desperation, he retreated to his grandfather's cabin in Montana, expecting to die.

Instead, something unexpected occurred. Removed from medical facilities, expert opinions, and treatment options, Michael was forced to listen to the one information source he had systematically ignored: his own body's intelligence.

"For decades, I treated my body like occupied territory requiring external governance," he later reflected. "In that cabin, I finally recognized it as the homeland I had been fighting to defend all along."

This revelation—that your body possesses intelligence vastly exceeding your conscious strategic planning—represents the oracle's bargain. Trading the illusion of control for partnership with inherent biological wisdom isn't surrender to disease but alignment with the most sophisticated healing system evolution has produced.

Research increasingly confirms this counterintuitive principle. Studies of the placebo effect reveal that belief in treatment activates identical neurobiological pathways as medical interventions. The emerging field of psychoneuroimmunology demonstrates that conscious attention itself directly modulates immune function, enhancing or suppressing inflammatory responses through pathways science is only beginning to understand.

The health strategist who masters partnership with these inherent mechanisms achieves what external intervention alone cannot: coordination with healing intelligence that precedes and will outlast all medical systems.

The Hospice Paradox

Perhaps the most heretical evidence against the warfare model of health comes from an unexpected source: hospice care. Medical professionals consistently report a puzzling phenomenon—patients who, after discontinuing aggressive treatments and accepting terminal prognoses, experience unexpected improvements and occasionally complete remissions.

This "hospice paradox" defies conventional explanation. Why would ceasing to fight disease sometimes lead to healing? The answer lies not in medicine but in strategy's deepest wisdom.

Sun Tzu wrote: "The supreme art of war is to subdue the enemy without fighting." In health terms, this manifests as the recognition that struggling against symptoms often strengthens the very processes creating them. The nervous system interprets battle orientation as threat, triggering cascades of stress hormones that inhibit regenerative function. The immune system, responding to psychological distress, prioritizes acute defense over chronic repair.

The hospice patient, paradoxically accepting mortality, often releases this counterproductive struggle. Their nervous system shifts from fight-or-flight to rest-and-repair. Their endocrine system reallocates resources from emergency response to foundational maintenance. Their psychology transitions from resistance to acceptance, eliminating a primary source of physiological burden.

This isn't magical thinking but strategic brilliance. As one oncologist observed: "Sometimes the most aggressive treatment is gentle surrender."

The Strategic Embrace

If warfare provides an incomplete metaphor for health, what alternative framework might better serve? Consider the strategic embrace—the capacity to fully encounter reality rather than battle against it.

Sarah discovered this approach through necessity after conventional treatments failed her multiple sclerosis. Rather than escalating the fight, she radically shifted orientation. She began systematically exploring her condition—not as enemy to be vanquished but as territory to be intimately known.

She documented precisely which foods triggered neurological symptoms. She mapped exactly how stress patterns preceded flares. She cataloged which environments supported function and which degraded capacity. She measured how specific sleep qualities predicted next-day ability.

"I stopped trying to defeat MS," Sarah explained, "and instead became a cartographer of my condition. The territory didn't change, but my relationship to it transformed completely."

This strategic embrace—studying reality with precision rather than struggling against it with force—yielded unexpected results. Within eighteen months, Sarah's disease progression halted. Within three years, many symptoms reversed. Not through conquest but through intimate knowledge that enabled strategic positioning.

The ancient Taoist principle applies perfectly: "To know others is intelligence; to know yourself is wisdom." The health strategist who masters this distinction transcends the limitations of both conventional and alternative medicine by recognizing that intimate self-knowledge provides strategic advantage no external system can match.

Beyond the Battlefield

The ultimate heresy awaiting the health warrior is this: your body was never a battlefield in the first place.

The military metaphor, while occasionally useful, fundamentally distorts biological reality. Cancer cells aren't invading enemies but your own tissues responding to signals you unconsciously provide. Autoimmune conditions aren't rebellions but communication systems seeking attention through increasingly desperate measures. Chronic inflammation isn't friendly fire but the body's attempt to address persistent threats it cannot eliminate.

This perspective shift—from battlefield to ecosystem, from occupation to membership, from warfare to governance—transforms everything. The symptoms that appeared as attacks reveal themselves as messages. The interventions previously deployed as weaponry become instead diplomatic communications. The struggle that felt like existential warfare transforms into skillful stewardship.

James, recovering from traumatic brain injury, expressed this revelation perfectly: "I spent months at war with my brain's limitations until I realized something obvious—my brain wasn't trying to limit me; it was trying to heal me according to principles I didn't understand."

By studying the patterns of his cognitive function with curious attention rather than frustrated resistance, James discovered something remarkable—his brain functioned brilliantly in specific circumstances while struggling in others. By arranging his life to leverage these patterns rather than fighting against them, he achieved more functional recovery than specialists predicted possible.

This represents strategy in its highest form—not imposing will upon reality but aligning action with existing patterns to achieve objectives that force alone cannot accomplish.

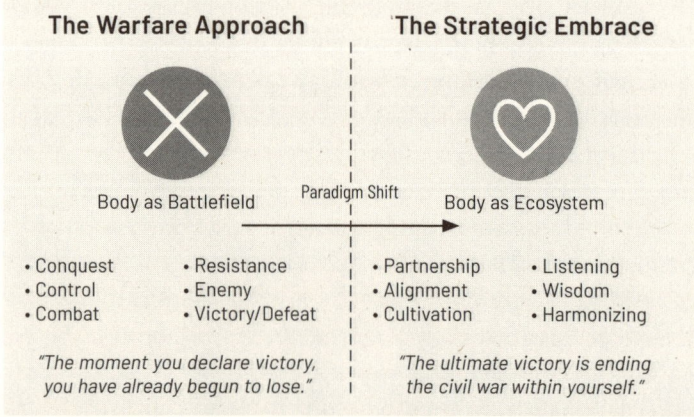

The Final Surrender

As you close this book and continue your health journey, consider the possibility that genuine strategy may require surrendering the very framework that brought you to these pages.

The war metaphor served its purpose—it mobilized resources, focused attention, and organized action when you needed those functions most. Like all models, however, it contains inherent limitations that eventually become constraints. The most sophisticated strategist recognizes when familiar frameworks have served their purpose and must be transcended.

What might health look like beyond warfare? Perhaps it resembles gardening more than combat—cultivating conditions where vitality naturally flourishes rather than battling endlessly against disorder. Perhaps it resembles diplomacy more than conquest—establishing beneficial relationships with the trillions of organisms comprising your microbiome rather than attempting to control them. Perhaps it resembles ecosystem management more than territorial defense—supporting natural cycles of regeneration rather than imposing arbitrary stability.

The health journey that begins with war strategy paradoxically concludes with the recognition that the most powerful strategy may be transcending strategy itself—moving from calculated intervention to aligned participation with the intelligent systems already operating within you.

Your body isn't enemy territory to be conquered, allied ground to be defended, or even neutral space to be governed. It is you—not metaphorically but literally. The ultimate victory isn't winning a war against disease but ending the civil war within yourself—the endless struggle between who you are and who you think you should be.

In that surrender lies the only victory that truly matters.

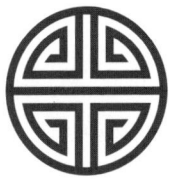

Author's Notes

Introduction

1. The individuals whose stories appear throughout this book represent composite cases drawn from research, observations, and common health patterns. Names and specific details have been created to illustrate strategic principles while protecting privacy. These examples demonstrate possible applications of the concepts discussed but do not guarantee similar results for any individual reader. This book presents strategic frameworks for understanding health, not specific medical protocols. Always consult qualified healthcare providers before modifying treatments, medications, or health routines, especially if you have existing medical conditions.

Chapter 1

1. This risk estimate is based on findings from the Framingham Heart Study, which found that having a first-degree relative with premature coronary heart disease increases risk by 2–3

fold (Lloyd-Jones et al., 2004). Lloyd-Jones, D. M., Nam, B. H., D'Agostino, R. B., Levy, D., Murabito, J. M., Wang, T. J., Wilson, P. W., & O'Donnell, C. J. (2004). "Parental cardiovascular disease as a risk factor for cardiovascular disease in middle-aged adults: a prospective study of parents and offspring." *JAMA*, 291(18), 2204–2211.

2. This figure is derived from a meta-analysis by Nicholson et al. (2006) that examined the association between depression and coronary heart disease. Nicholson, A., Kuper, H., & Hemingway, H. (2006). "Depression as an aetiologic and prognostic factor in coronary heart disease: a meta-analysis of 6,362 events among 146,538 participants in 54 observational studies." *European Heart Journal*, 27(23), 2763–2774.

3. This finding is based on research by Ryan & Deci (2000) on Self-Determination Theory, which demonstrates that autonomously motivated behaviors (those aligned with personal values) show significantly higher adherence rates than externally motivated ones. Ryan, R. M., & Deci, E. L. (2000). "Self-determination theory and the facilitation of intrinsic motivation, social development, and well-being." *American Psychologist*, 55(1), 68–78.

4. A meta-analysis by Nussbaumer-Streit et al. (2021) found that light therapy showed efficacy comparable to antidepressant medication for seasonal affective disorder. Nussbaumer-Streit, B., Thaler, K., Chapman, A., Probst, T., Winkler, D., Sönnichsen, A., Gaynes, B. N., & Gartlehner, G. (2021). Second-generation antidepressants for treatment of seasonal affective disorder. The Cochrane database of systematic reviews, 3(3), CD008591.

5. This data is drawn from research by Barton et al. (2013) on supporting targeted hip/ gluteal strengthening in PFPS. Barton, C. J., Lack, S., Malliaras, P., & Morrissey, D. (2013). "Gluteal muscle activity and patellofemoral pain syndrome:

a systematic review." *British Journal of Sports Medicine*, 47(4), 207–214.
6. Han's 2024 research is a leading source for this evidence-based conclusion, with corroborating findings in broader literature on shift work, health adaptation, and personalized routines. Han W. J. (2024). How our longitudinal employment patterns might shape our health as we approach middle adulthood-US NLSY79 cohort. PloS one, 19(4), e0300245.
7. This refers to research by Wing & Phelan (2005) on long-term weight management, which found that individuals making moderate, sustainable changes maintained improvements longer than those using more extreme approaches. Wing, R. R., & Phelan, S. (2005). "Long-term weight loss maintenance." *The American Journal of Clinical Nutrition*, 82(1), 222S–225S.

Chapter 2
1. Return on investment data from Masters, R., et al. (2017). "Return on investment of public health interventions: A systematic review." *Journal of Epidemiology & Community Health*, 71(8), 827–834.
2. This statistic comes from Allegrante, J. P., Wells, M. T., & Peterson, J. C. (2019). "Interventions to support behavioral self-management of chronic diseases." *Annual Review of Public Health*, 40(1), 127–146.
3. Cost figures derived from American Diabetes Association. (2024). "Economic costs of diabetes." Diabetes Care, 47(1); American Heart Association. (2023). "Heart disease and stroke statistics." *Circulation*, 147(8); National Cancer Institute. (2022). "Financial burden of cancer care."
4. Breast cancer treatment costs from Blumen, H., Fitch, K., & Polkus, V. (2016). "Comparison of treatment costs for breast cancer, by tumor stage and type of service." American health & drug benefits, 9(1), 23.

5. While these figures are estimates and depend on individual circumstances, the evidence consistently supports the substantial health and economic benefits of regular physical activity like walking. Walking benefits quantified based on Lee, I.M., et al. (2022). "Association of step volume and intensity with all-cause mortality." *JAMA Internal Medicine*, 182(11), 1139-1148; Kraus, W.E., et al. (2023). "Physical activity and health: Updated recommendation." *American Journal of Preventive Medicine*, 65(2).
6. While these figures are estimates and depend on individual circumstances, the evidence consistently supports the substantial health and economic benefits of a Mediterranean diet. Mediterranean diet benefits based on meta-analyses by Dinu, M., Pagliai, G., Casini, A., & Sofi, F. (2018). "Mediterranean diet and multiple health outcomes: an umbrella review of meta-analyses of observational studies and randomised trials." *European Journal of Clinical Nutrition*, 72(1), 30–43.
7. While these figures are estimates and depend on individual circumstances, the evidence consistently supports the substantial health, cognitive, and economic benefits of prioritizing quality sleep.
8. Diabetes progression costs adapted from Herman, W. H. (2011). "The economics of diabetes prevention." *Medical Clinics*, 95(2), 373–384.
9. The "13% more productive" figure comes from a field study of British Telecom call-center workers that links weekly self-reported happiness to sales and finds ~13% higher sales in happier weeks (later published in *Management Science*). The "25% more likely to have high job performance" and "27% lower absenteeism" figures come from a *Journal of Occupational and Environmental Medicine* study of 20,114 U.S. employees using the Healthways Well-Being Assessment.

Chapter 3

1. These estimates are supported by the World Cancer Research Fund and American Institute for Cancer Research (2018). "Diet, nutrition, physical activity and cancer: A global perspective." *The Third Expert Report.*
2. Based on findings from the Diabetes Prevention Program Research Group (2002). "Reduction in the incidence of type 2 diabetes with lifestyle intervention or metformin." *New England Journal of Medicine*, 346(6), 393–403.
3. For current BRCA1 risk statistics, see Kuchenbaecker, K. B., et al. (2017). "Risks of breast, ovarian, and contralateral breast cancer for BRCA1 and BRCA2 mutation carriers." *JAMA*, 317(23), 2402–2416.
4. Sutton, E. F., et al. (2018). "Early time-restricted feeding improves insulin sensitivity, blood pressure, and oxidative stress even without weight loss in men with prediabetes." *Cell Metabolism*, 27(6), 1212-1221.
5. de Groot, S., et al. (2020). "Fasting mimicking diet as an adjunct to neoadjuvant chemotherapy for breast cancer in the multicentre randomized phase 2 DIRECT trial." *Nature Communications*, 11, 3083.
6. Dimitrova, A. K., et al. (2013). "Prevalence of migraine in patients with celiac disease and inflammatory bowel disease." *Headache*, 53(2), 344–355.
7. Sachdeva, A., et al. (2009). "Lipid levels in patients hospitalized with coronary artery disease: An analysis of 136,905 hospitalizations in Get With The Guidelines." *American Heart Journal*, 157(1), 111-117.
8. Hibbard, J. H., & Greene, J. (2013). "What the evidence shows about patient activation: Better health outcomes and care experiences; fewer data on costs. *Health Affairs*, 32(2), 207–214.

Chapter 4

1. Hancock, K., et al. (2009). "Cross-reactive antibody responses to the 2009 pandemic H1N1 influenza virus." *Nature Immunology*, 10(12), 1221–1227.
2. Stampfer, M. J., Hu, F. B., Manson, J. E., Rimm, E. B., & Willett, W. C. (2000). "Primary prevention of coronary heart disease in women through diet and lifestyle." *New England Journal of Medicine*, 343(1), 16–22.
3. Centers for Medicare & Medicaid Services. (2022). National Health Expenditure Data. https://www.cms.gov/Research-Statistics-Data-and-Systems/Statistics-Trends-and-Reports/NationalHealthExpendData
4. World Health Organization. (2018). "Noncommunicable diseases country profiles 2018." Geneva: World Health Organization.
5. Goodpaster, B. H., & Sparks, L. M. (2017). "Metabolic flexibility in health and disease." *Cell Metabolism*, 25(5), 1027–1036.
6. Shaffer, F., & Ginsberg, J. P. (2017). "An overview of heart rate variability metrics and norms." *Frontiers in Public Health*, 5, 258.
7. Prüss-Üstün, A., Wolf, J., Corvalán, C., Bos, R., & Neira, M. (2016). "Preventing disease through healthy environments: A global assessment of the burden of disease from environmental risks." World Health Organization.
8. Buettner, D., & Skemp, S. (2016). "Blue Zones: Lessons from the world's longest lived." *American Journal of Lifestyle Medicine*, 10(5), 318–321.
9. Waldinger, R. J., & Schulz, M. S. (2010). "What's love got to do with it? Social functioning, perceived health, and daily happiness in married octogenarians." *Journal of Happiness Studies*, 11(1), 71–89.
10. Mattson, M. P. (2008). Hormesis defined. *Ageing Research Reviews*, 7(1), 1–7.

Chapter 5

1. The energy management research referenced here comes from Schwartz and McCarthy's (2007) work "Manage Your Energy, Not Your Time" published in *Harvard Business Review*, which identified four dimensions of energy that require management: physical, emotional, mental, and spiritual.

2. Wing and Phelan (2005) reviewed multiple studies on weight loss maintenance and found that approximately 80% of individuals who lose weight regain it within a year, supporting the notion that conventional approaches to behavior change often fail to produce sustainable results.

3. Ames (2006) proposed the triage theory of micronutrient deficiency in the Proceedings of the National Academy of Sciences, suggesting that chronic, low-level deficiencies in essential nutrients prioritize short-term survival at the expense of long-term health, creating cellular energy deficits even in the absence of clinical deficiency symptoms.

4. The American Psychological Association's annual "Stress in America" survey (2021) has consistently shown high levels of stress affecting health behaviors, with pandemic-related stressors exacerbating pre-existing trends of stress-related health behavior deterioration.

5. Christakis and Fowler's (2007) landmark study published in the *New England Journal of Medicine* tracked over 12,000 people for 32 years and found that having an obese friend increased one's chance of obesity by 57%, demonstrating the powerful influence of social networks on health behaviors.

6. Cohen et al. (2016) conducted a meta-analysis published in *Psychosomatic Medicine* that found a significant association between purpose in life and reduced all-cause mortality and cardiovascular events, independent of other psychological variables.

7. Fisher et al. (2017) published findings in *Experimental Gerontology* demonstrating that multiple daily sets of resistance exer-

cise distributed throughout the day produced similar strength gains to the same volume performed in a single session, while improving adherence in previously sedentary adults.
8. The cascade effect described here is supported by Mata et al. (2009), who found in a study published in *Psychology of Sport and Exercise* that successful exercise engagement predicted subsequent improvement in eating regulation, suggesting that strategically timed physical activity can trigger positive behavioral cascades.
9. World Health Organization (2018). The top 10 causes of death. WHO fact sheets detail that noncommunicable diseases account for 71% of global deaths, with a significant portion preventable through lifestyle modification targeting common risk factors.

Chapter 6

1. Boersma, P., Black, L. I., & Ward, B. W. (2020). Prevalence of Multiple Chronic Conditions Among US Adults, 2018. *Preventing Chronic Disease*, 17, E106.
2. Rappaport, S. M. (2016). "Genetic factors are not the major causes of chronic diseases." *PLOS ONE*, 11(4), e0154387.
3. Nation, D. A., Sweeney, M. D., Montagne, A., Sagare, A. P., D'Orazio, L. M., Pachicano, M., ... & Zlokovic, B. V. (2019). "Blood-brain barrier breakdown is an early biomarker of human cognitive dysfunction." *Nature Medicine*, 25(2), 270–276.
4. Irwin, M. R., Olmstead, R., & Carroll, J. E. (2016). "Sleep Disturbance, Sleep Duration, and Inflammation: A Systematic Review and Meta-Analysis of Cohort Studies and Experimental Sleep Deprivation." *Biological Psychiatry*, 80(1), 40–52.
5. Cohen, S., Janicki-Deverts, D., Doyle, W. J., Miller, G. E., Frank, E., Rabin, B. S., & Turner, R. B. (2012). "Chronic stress, glucocorticoid receptor resistance, inflammation, and disease risk." Proceedings of the National Academy of Sci-

ences of the United States of America, 109(16), 5995–5999.
6. Black, D. S., & Slavich, G. M. (2016). "Mindfulness meditation and the immune system: a systematic review of randomized controlled trials." *Annals of the New York Academy of Sciences*, 1373(1), 13–24.
7. Arnsten A. F. (2015). "Stress weakens prefrontal networks: molecular insults to higher cognition." *Nature Neuroscience*, 18(10), 1376–1385.
8. Ridker P. M. (2014). "LDL cholesterol: controversies and future therapeutic directions." *Lancet* (London, England), 384(9943), 607–617.
9. Hafdi, M., Hoevenaar-Blom, M. P., & Richard, E. (2021). "Multi-domain interventions for the prevention of dementia and cognitive decline." The Cochrane database of systematic reviews, 11(11), CD013572.

Chapter 7

1. Statistics from Centers for Disease Control and Prevention. (2022). Chronic diseases in America. Retrieved from CDC.gov. Current data indicates these percentages have risen since publication.
2. World Health Organization. (2023). Noncommunicable diseases fact sheet. WHO Global Health Observatory.
3. Li, Y., Pan, A., Wang, D.D., et al. (2018). "Impact of healthy lifestyle factors on life expectancies in the US population." *Circulation*, 138(4), 345–355.
4. Cavero-Redondo, I., Martinez-Vizcaino, V., Fernandez-Rodriguez, R., Saz-Lara, A., Pascual-Morena, C., & Álvarez-Bueno, C. (2020). "Effect of Behavioral Weight Management Interventions Using Lifestyle mHealth Self-Monitoring on Weight Loss: A Systematic Review and Meta-Analysis." *Nutrients*, 12(7), 1977.
5. Melamed, S., Shirom, A., Toker, S., Berliner, S., & Shapira, I.

(2006). "Burnout and risk of cardiovascular disease: evidence, possible causal paths, and promising research directions." *Psychological Bulletin*, 132(3), 327–353.
6. Saver J. L. (2006). "Time is brain—quantified." *Stroke*, 37(1), 263–266.
7. Wood, W., & Neal, D.T. (2016). "Healthy through habit: Interventions for initiating & maintaining health behavior change." *Behavioral Science & Policy*, 2(1), 71-83.
8. Hall, K.D., Ayuketah, A., Brychta, R., et al. (2019). Ultra-processed diets cause excess calorie intake and weight gain. *Cell Metabolism*, 30(1), 67–77.e3.
9. Thomas, J. G., Bond, D. S., Phelan, S., Hill, J. O., & Wing, R. R. (2014). "Weight-loss maintenance for 10 years in the National Weight Control Registry." *American Journal of Preventive Medicine*, 46(1), 17–23.
10. Christakis, N. A., & Fowler, J. H. (2007). "The spread of obesity in a large social network over 32 years." *The New England Journal of Medicine*, 357(4), 370–379.

Chapter 8

1. The American Heart Association's Life's Essential 8 metrics now include sleep health as a critical component, expanding from the previous Simple 7 framework. For full details, see Lloyd-Jones et al. (2022). Life's Essential 8: Updating and enhancing the American Heart Association's construct of cardiovascular health. *Circulation*, 146(5), e18–e28.
2. This references the Global Burden of Disease study published in *The Lancet*. See GBD 2017 Diet Collaborators. (2019). "Health effects of dietary risks in 195 countries, 1990-2017: A systematic analysis for the Global Burden of Disease Study 2017." *The Lancet*, 393(10184), 1958–1972.
3. For more on the gut-brain axis and serotonin production, see Yano et al. (2015). "Indigenous bacteria from the gut microbi-

ota regulate host serotonin biosynthesis." *Cell*, 161(2), 264–276.
4. This refers to the groundbreaking personalized nutrition study by Zeevi et al. (2015). "Personalized nutrition by prediction of glycemic responses." *Cell*, 163(5), 1079–1094.
5. This statistic comes from Prasad et al. (2013). "A decade of reversal: An analysis of 146 contradicted medical practices." *Mayo Clinic Proceedings*, 88(8), 790–798.
6. For a comprehensive guide to evaluating medical evidence, see Ebell et al. (2004). "Strength of recommendation taxonomy (SORT): A patient-centered approach to grading evidence in the medical literature." *American Family Physician*, 69(3), 548–556.
7. FODMAP (Fermentable Oligosaccharides, Disaccharides, Monosaccharides, and Polyols) refers to poorly absorbed carbs that can cause digestive issues like bloating. A low-FODMAP diet reduces these carbs to help manage symptoms, especially in people with IBS.
8. For more on exercise periodization, see Kiely, J. (2018). "Periodization theory: Confronting an inconvenient truth." *Sports Medicine*, 48(4), 753–764.
9. The WHO's shift to "adaptive aging" is detailed in World Health Organization. (2017). Global strategy and action plan on ageing and health. Geneva: World Health Organization.

Chapter 9

1. World Health Organization. (2022). Physical inactivity: A global public health problem. Global Strategy on Diet, Physical Activity and Health. Statistics updated annually; figures represent most recent global assessment.
2. Veerman, J. L., Healy, G. N., Cobiac, L. J., Vos, T., Winkler, E. A., Owen, N., & Dunstan, D. W. (2012). "Television viewing time and reduced life expectancy: A life table analysis." *British Journal of Sports Medicine*, 46(13), 927–930.

3. Owen, N., Sparling, P. B., Healy, G. N., Dunstan, D. W., & Matthews, C. E. (2010, December). "Sedentary behavior: emerging evidence for a new health risk." In *Mayo Clinic Proceedings* (Vol. 85, No. 12, p. 1138).
4. Coates, A. M., Joyner, M. J., Little, J. P., Jones, A. M., & Gibala, M. J. (2023). "A perspective on high-intensity interval training for performance and health." *Sports Medicine*, 53(Suppl 1), 85–96. This research demonstrates specific cellular mechanisms activated by brief, intense exercise.
5. Katzmarzyk, P. T., Powell, K. E., & Jakicic, J. M. (2019). "Sedentary behavior and health: Update from the 2018 Physical Activity Guidelines Advisory Committee." *Medicine & Science in Sports & Exercise*, 51(6), 1227–1241.
6. Florence, C. S., Bergen, G., Atherly, A., Burns, E., Stevens, J., & Drake, C. (2018). "Medical costs of fatal and nonfatal falls in older adults." *Journal of the American Geriatrics Society*, 66(4), 693–698. Fall prevention represents one of healthcare's highest-value interventions.
7. Sato, S., Basse, A. L., Schönke, M., Chen, S., Samad, M., Altıntaş, A., … & Sassone-Corsi, P. (2019). "Time of exercise specifies the impact on muscle metabolic pathways and systemic energy homeostasis." *Cell Metabolism*, 30(1), 92–110.
8. Vargas-Molina, S., Petro, J. L., Romance, R., Bonilla, D. A., Schoenfeld, B. J., Kreider, R. B., & Benítez-Porres, J. (2022). "Menstrual cycle-based undulating periodized program effects on body composition and strength in trained women: a pilot study." *Science & Sports*, 37(8), 753–761.
9. Centers for Disease Control and Prevention. (2023). Physical Activity Guidelines for Americans compliance report. National Center for Health Statistics Data Brief, No. 443. Despite decades of public education, adherence remains a primary public health challenge.
10. Manini, T. M., & Pahor, M. (2009). "Physical activity and

maintaining physical function in older adults." *British Journal of Sports Medicine*, 43(1), 28–31.

Chapter 10

1. Research by Sternfeld et al. (2014) showed that regular exercise significantly reduced menopausal symptoms, while mindfulness-based stress reduction demonstrated comparable effects in a randomized controlled trial by Carmody et al. (2011).
2. See Cohen et al. (2019) for a comprehensive meta-analysis on the physiological pathways connecting chronic stress to major disease pathology.
3. Holt-Lunstad et al. (2010) conducted a meta-analysis of 148 studies finding that strong social relationships increased survival likelihood by 50%, comparable to quitting smoking.
4. Vaillant, G. E. (2012). Triumphs of experience: The men of the Harvard Grant Study. Harvard University Press. This 75+ year study remains the gold standard for understanding factors affecting healthy aging.
5. Metaanalysis by Peterson et al. (2011) in *Medicine & Science in Sports & Exercise* demonstrated significant reversal of sarcopenia through progressive resistance training across age groups.
6. The CDC's STEADI (Stopping Elderly Accidents, Deaths & Injuries) program synthesizes evidence-based approaches to fall prevention with demonstrated efficacy across diverse populations (Burns et al., 2016).
7. The FINGER study (Ngandu et al., 2015) demonstrated that multimodal interventions including cognitive training reduced dementia risk by 30–47% in at-risk populations.
8. Makary & Daniel (2016) analysis in *BMJ* concluded that medical errors account for more than 250,000 deaths annually, making them the third leading cause of death after heart disease and cancer.
9. Hibbard & Greene (2013) demonstrated in *Health Affairs* that

activated patients who participate in care coordination show significantly better health outcomes and care experiences.
10. See Neff & Germer (2017) for an overview of how self-compassion practices improve health behaviors and outcomes across numerous clinical populations.

Chapter 11

1. Centers for Disease Control and Prevention. (2023). *National Diabetes Statistics Report*. Atlanta, GA: Centers for Disease Control and Prevention, U.S. Department of Health and Human Services.
2. Besedovsky, L., Lange, T., & Born, J. (2012). "Sleep and immune function." *Pflügers Archiv—European Journal of Physiology*, 463(1), 121–137.
3. Rondanelli, M., et al. (2018). "Self-care for common colds: The pivotal role of vitamin D, vitamin C, zinc, and Echinacea in three main immune interactive clusters." *Evidence-Based Complementary and Alternative Medicine*, 2018, 5813095.
4. Mainous, A. G., Tanner, R. J., & Baker, R. (2016). "Prediabetes diagnosis and treatment in primary care." *Journal of the American Board of Family Medicine*, 29(2), 283–285.
5. Turati, F., Carioli, G., Bravi, F., Ferraroni, M., Serraino, D., Montella, M., ... & La Vecchia, C. (2018). "Mediterranean diet and breast cancer risk." *Nutrients*, 10(3), 326.
6. Sedaghat, F., et al. (2016). "Mediterranean diet adherence and risk of multiple sclerosis: a case-control study." *Asia Pacific Journal of Clinical Nutrition*, 25(2), 377-384.
7. Rains, J. C., Poceta, J. S., & Penzien, D. B. (2008). "Sleep and headaches." *Current Neurology and Neuroscience Reports*, 8(2), 167–175.
8. Liu, Y., et al. (2016). Clustering of five health-related behaviors for chronic disease prevention among adults, United States, 2013. Preventing Chronic Disease, 13, E70.

9. Cormie, P., Zopf, E. M., Zhang, X., & Schmitz, K. H. (2017). "The impact of exercise on cancer mortality, recurrence, and treatment-related adverse effects." *Epidemiologic Reviews*, 39(1), 71–92.

Chapter 12

1. Centers for Disease Control and Prevention. (2023). Chronic diseases in America. National Center for Chronic Disease Prevention and Health Promotion.
2. Finckh, A., Liang, M. H., van Herckenrode, C. M., & de Pablo, P. (2006). "Long-term impact of early treatment on radiographic progression in rheumatoid arthritis: A meta-analysis." *Arthritis & Rheumatism*, 55(6), 864–872.
3. World Health Organization. (2023). Global initiative for emergency and essential surgical care. WHO Surgical Care Systems Strengthening Program.
4. Wilmott, J. S., Scolyer, R. A., Long, G. V., & Hersey, P. (2012). "Combined targeted therapy and immunotherapy in the treatment of advanced melanoma." *Oncoimmunology*, 1(6), 997–999.
5. Hallberg, S. J., McKenzie, A. L., Williams, P. T., Bhanpuri, N. H., Peters, A. L., Campbell, W. W., Hazbun, T. L., Volk, B. M., McCarter, J. P., Phinney, S. D., & Volek, J. S. (2018). "Effectiveness and Safety of a Novel Care Model for the Management of Type 2 Diabetes at 1 Year: An Open-Label, Non-Randomized, Controlled Study." Diabetes therapy: research, treatment and education of diabetes and related disorders, 9(2), 583–612.
6. Ornish, D., Scherwitz, L. W., Billings, J. H., Brown, S. E., Gould, K. L., Merritt, T. A., Sparler, S., Armstrong, W. T., Ports, T. A., Kirkeeide, R. L., Hogeboom, C., & Brand, R. J. (1998). "Intensive lifestyle changes for reversal of coronary heart disease." *JAMA*, 280(23), 2001–2007.
7. Muraro, P. A., Pasquini, M., Atkins, H. L., Bowen, J. D.,

Farge, D., Fassas, A., Freedman, M. S., Georges, G. E., Gualandi, F., Hamerschlak, N., Havrdova, E., Kimiskidis, V. K., Kozak, T., Mancardi, G. L., Massacesi, L., Moraes, D. A., Nash, R. A., Pavletic, S., Ouyang, J., Rovira, M., ... "Multiple Sclerosis–Autologous Hematopoietic Stem Cell Transplantation (MS-AHSCT) Long-term Outcomes Study Group (2017). Long-term Outcomes After Autologous Hematopoietic Stem Cell Transplantation for Multiple Sclerosis." *JAMA Neurology*, 74(4), 459–469.

8. Garland, E. L., Hanley, A. W., Nakamura, Y., Barrett, J. W., Baker, A. K., Reese, S. E., Riquino, M. R., Froeliger, B., & Donaldson, G. W. (2022). "Mindfulness-Oriented Recovery Enhancement vs Supportive Group Therapy for Co-occurring Opioid Misuse and Chronic Pain in Primary Care: A Randomized Clinical Trial." *JAMA Internal Medicine*, 182(4), 407–417.

9. Moyer, R., Ikert, K., Long, K., & Marsh, J. (2017). "The Value of Preoperative Exercise and Education for Patients Undergoing Total Hip and Knee Arthroplasty: A Systematic Review and Meta-Analysis." *JBJS reviews*, 5(12), e2.

10. Anand, P., Kunnumakkara, A. B., Sundaram, C., Harikumar, K. B., Tharakan, S. T., Lai, O. S., Sung, B., & Aggarwal, B. B. (2008). "Cancer is a preventable disease that requires major lifestyle changes." Pharmaceutical research, 25(9), 2097–2116.

Chapter 13

1. These statistics are from Magnusson, R. (2019). *Non-Communicable Diseases and Global Health Politics*. The Oxford Handbook of Global Health Politics.
2. Based on research by Safer, M. A., Tharps, Q. J., Jackson, T. C., & Leventhal, H. (1979). "Determinants of three stages of delay in seeking care at a medical clinic." *Medical Care*, 17(1), 11–29.

3. Market projection from Grand View Research (2023). Health wearable market size report, 2023–2030.
4. Shcherbina, A., Mattsson, C. M., Waggott, D., Salisbury, H., Christle, J. W., Hastie, T., Wheeler, M. T., & Ashley, E. A. (2017). "Accuracy in Wrist-Worn, Sensor-Based Measurements of Heart Rate and Energy Expenditure in a Diverse Cohort." *Journal of Personalized Medicine*, 7(2), 3.
5. McAndrew, L. M., Phillips, L. A., Helmer, D. A., Maestro, K., Engel, C. C., Greenberg, L. M., Anastasides, N., & Quigley, K. S. (2017). "High healthcare utilization near the onset of medically unexplained symptoms." *Journal of Psychosomatic Research*, 98, 98–105.
6. Amawi, R. M., & Murdoch, M. J. (2022). "Effects of pill colors on human perception and expectation of drugs' efficacy." *Color Research & Application*, 47(5), 1200–1215.
7. Hibbard, J. H., & Greene, J. (2013). "What the evidence shows about patient activation: better health outcomes and care experiences; fewer data on costs." *Health Affairs*, 32(2), 207–214.
8. Waldinger, R. J., & Schulz, M. S. (2023). *The Good Life: Lessons from the World's Longest Scientific Study of Happiness*. Simon & Schuster.
9. Allen, J. G., MacNaughton, P., Satish, U., Santanam, S., Vallarino, J., & Spengler, J. D. (2016). Associations of Cognitive Function Scores with Carbon Dioxide, Ventilation, and Volatile Organic Compound Exposures in Office Workers: A Controlled Exposure Study of Green and Conventional Office Environments. Environmental health perspectives, 124(6), 805–812.
10. Shetty, S., & Mahale, A. (2022). "Comprehensive Review of Multimodal Medical data Analysis: open issues and future research Directions." *Acta Informatica Pragensia*, 11(3), 423–457.

"Books to Span the East and West"

Tuttle Publishing was founded in 1832 in the small New England town of Rutland, Vermont [USA]. Our core values remain as strong today as they were then—to publish best-in-class books which bring people together one page at a time. In 1948, we established a publishing outpost in Japan—and Tuttle is now a leader in publishing English-language books about the arts, languages and cultures of Asia. The world has become a much smaller place today and Asia's economic and cultural influence has grown. Yet the need for meaningful dialogue and information about this diverse region has never been greater. Over the past seven decades, Tuttle has published thousands of books on subjects ranging from martial arts and paper crafts to language learning and literature—and our talented authors, illustrators, designers and photographers have won many prestigious awards. We welcome you to explore the wealth of information available on Asia at **www.tuttlepublishing.com**.

First published by Tuttle Publishing, an imprint of Periplus Editions (HK) Ltd.

www.tuttlepublishing.com

Copyright © 2026 Y. Tony Yang

All rights reserved. No part of this publication may be reproduced or utilized in any form or by any means, electronic or mechanical, including photocopying, recording, or by any information storage and retrieval system, without prior written permission from the publisher.

Library of Congress Catalog-in-Publication Data in progress

ISBN: 978-0-8048-5858-8

29 28 27 26 25
10 9 8 7 6 5 4 3 2 1   2510VP

Printed in Malaysia

GPSR Representative
Matt Parsons, matt.parsons@upi2mbooks.hr
UPI-2M PLUS d.o.o., Medulićeva 20
10000 Zagreb, Croatia

Distributed by:

North America, Latin America & Europe
Tuttle Publishing
364 Innovation Drive
North Clarendon
VT 05759 9436, USA
Tel: 1(802) 773 8930
Fax: 1(802) 773 6993
info@tuttlepublishing.com
www.tuttlepublishing.com

Asia Pacific
Berkeley Books Pte Ltd
3 Kallang Sector #04-01
Singapore 349278
Tel: (65) 6741-2178
Fax: (65) 6741-2179
inquiries@periplus.com.sg
www.tuttlepublishing.com

Japan
Tuttle Publishing
Yaekari Building, 3rd Floor
5-4-12 Osaki Shinagawa-ku
Tokyo 141 0032 Japan
Tel: 81 (3) 5437 0171
Fax: 81 (3) 5437 0755
sales@tuttle.co.jp
www.tuttle.co.jp

TUTTLE PUBLISHING® is a registered trademark of Tuttle Publishing, a division of Periplus Editions (HK) Ltd.